6/72

THE NEUROLOGICAL EXAMINATION OF THE CHILD WITH MINOR NERVOUS DYSFUNCTION

Clinics in Developmental Medicine No. 38

The Neurological Examination
of the Child with
Minor Nervous Dysfunction

BERT C. L. TOUWEN
HEINZ F. R. PRECHTL

Department of Developmental Neurology,
University Hospital, Groningen,
The Netherlands.

Spastics International Medical Publications

LONDON: William Heinemann Medical Books Ltd.

PHILADELPHIA: J. B. Lippincott Co.

SBN 433-32620-4

Printed in England at THE LAVENHAM PRESS LTD., Lavenham, Suffolk.

Contents

ACKNOWLEDGEMENTS

Our thanks are due to A. F. Kalverboer, Ph.D., for his critical remarks, and to Dr. Martin C. O. Bax for his help in the preparation of the manuscript.

Our work was supported by a grant from Prinses Beatrix Fonds and the Organization for Health Research T.N.O.

Preface

Many workers, including Prechtl's own group in Groningen, have developed techniques for the examination of the nervous system of babies. The value of such work is undoubted, but its validation depends in part upon reliable neurological examinations of older children. In the course of their own follow-up studies, Touwen and Prechtl have become well aware of this problem and they present here a systematic method for examining the nervous system of the older child. It is not only for the purpose of follow-up studies of babies, however, that such a technique is necessary.

The classical neurological examination, developed largely in adults with overt disorders, is not an adequate tool for assessing the nervous system of the developing child. Yet the primary neurological training of most doctors is on adult patients, and it is perhaps not surprising that the neurological examination of the child is often unreliable. Even with supposedly familiar items such as the reflexes, colleagues and I have found that results showed wide variations, relating not to the different children examined but to the different doctors carrying out the examinations! Yet there is good evidence that there are many children with learning and/or behaviour difficulties who do have minor neurological dysfunction which requires exact and reliable assessment.

The first need in studying these children is the development of a reliable tool. Those familiar with the studies which Prechtl and his co-workers have made on babies will recognise in this book the same meticulous attention to detail that characterised their previous work. Each test is clearly described and illustrated and a pro-forma allows the results to be recorded in a manner which is readily quantifiable. With this tool, the physician is equipped to study the child with minor neurological dysfunction, in addition to assessing reliably those with major dysfunction.

MARTIN BAX

Foreword

The design of a rather extensive special neurological examination for children with only minor deviations in their neural functions requires some justification. Why are the ordinary neurological techniques employed by many neuropaediatricians and neurologists insufficient? The answer is relatively simple.

In many instances the children are selected for a full neurological examination because of complaints from parents and teachers of behavioural and/or learning difficulties. Often the children do not show any overt neurological symptoms or signs which could act as a guide for the strategy of the examination. Therefore the examination should be detailed and comprehensive, in order to assess a large variety of neural mechanisms. It is important not only that deviant signs should be identified, but also that the absence of deviant signs should be reliably confirmed. The classical neurological examination techniques are not sufficiently sensitive for this purpose. Because of their lack of quantification and strict standardization as regards methods, the state of the child, the sequence of tests, examination conditions, etc., they are too inaccurate for the specific problems we face with these children. A special method of neurological examination seems therefore to be justified. We believe that children who do have neurological deviations (and learning or behaviour problems) should be managed rather differently from children who do not have neurological signs but have learning or behaviour problems. This method can also be of value in the assessment of children with overt neurological handicaps, since it may reveal facets of their condition which will be significant for management, *e.g.* an overt hemiplegic may be found to have minor coordination difficulties in the 'normal' hand which require treatment.

But what, exactly, are the aims of such a refined technique? Obviously the neurological examination should detect functional defects or substantiate their absence. These should be clearly differentiated from deviations which stem from a lag in the speed of maturation of the brain: there are children with a mild retardation in the maturational process of their nervous system who show no indication of brain damage. The aim of a refined examination technique is to separate these cases, but not to supply a comprehensive developmental assessment, since standardized techniques have long been available for this purpose and the technique required is different from that for a neurological examination.

In any one item, such as the grasping of an object, a developmental assessment will give the child a score for the correct performance in accordance with the maturational time-table for that type of behaviour. The neurological examination, on the other hand, is concerned not only with whether or not the child performs the task but also with the way in which he performs the task. Some of the items in a neurological examination do, of course, show a developmental sequence and neurological deviation may account for a developmental delay. However, there are other causes of developmental delay which lie outside the central nervous system.

The neurological assessment belongs to the methodological arsenal of a new specialisation. As it is concerned with the most complex organ of the organism, it is not surprising that it involves comparably complex methods of examination which are difficult, time-consuming and require special skills and knowledge. This puts practical limits to the extent of the examination. All those functions for which specialists such as audiologists, ophthalmologists and speech therapists are already available, are excluded apart from a superficial screening. The assessment of vision, hearing and speech needs specialized techniques and any attempt to combine all the aspects within one examination would inevitably lead to imbalance in the thoroughness of the assessment: moreover, the assessments of visual and auditory acuity have been well described by other people so that these need not be repeated here.

It is unfortunate that no 'crucial' neurological tests can be identified to indicate whether the brain is functioning normally or abnormally. The plea for a short neurological screening, though understandable, ignores essential properties of the central nervous system. A neurological screening has many limitations in infants whose nervous system is relatively simple, and this applies even more in a study of the immensely more complex nervous system of the older child. In the future it may be possible to identify the most significant items in the neurological examination, but this is not possible at present. Examinations of any one aspect of the nervous system such as coordination may not give us any information about other aspects such as muscle power or reflexes. Within each aspect, two or three parameters must be studied, as we have little information about the significance of individual tests, and there is evidence that in some instances the correlation between them is not high. In addition, screening tests always run the risk of being mistaken for a proper examination, which they are not.

For over ten years at Groningen we have been following up groups of babies who were given very careful examinations in the neonatal period, and developing techniques for assessing the later neurological performance. There is a high correlation between newborn neurological deviation and signs at preschool age (Prechtl 1965). This present report describes what we now feel is the optimum tool for carrying out the neurological assessment of the child aged three to ten years. In many instances we have not yet been able to establish *accurate* population norms for tests, but we do have systematic data on many large groups of children. Statements about a developmental frequency of neurological performance are based on systematic examination of many hundreds of children and clinical assessment of many more.

Introduction

The existence of a syndrome of cerebral dysfunction, manifesting itself both in a neurological and a behavioural dimension, was first postulated by Goldstein (1936) and Strauss and Werner (1943). Since then, many papers on this subject have been published. Different authors have accentuated different aspects. The major symptom exhibited by children may be hyperactivity (Anderson 1963, Bakwin 1967, Eisenberg 1966, Ingram 1956, Millichap 1968, Minde *et al.* 1968, Sainz 1966, Stewart *et al.* 1966, Werry *et al.* 1964), clumsiness (Gubbay *et al.* 1965, Illingworth 1963, Reuben and Bakwin 1968, Walton 1963, Walton *et al.* 1962), visuomotor disabilities (Brenner *et al.* 1967, Walker 1965), delayed and/or irregular maturation (Abrams 1968, Illingworth 1968), or a high amount of associated movements (Abercrombie *et al.* 1964, Cohen *et al.* 1967, Connolly and Stratton 1968, Fog and Fog 1963, Zazzo 1960). Several reviews of these publications have attempted to define a specific syndrome (Bax and Mac Keith 1963; Clements 1962, 1966; Conners 1967; Pincus and Glaser 1966).

Unfortunately, a vague and global concept of minimal cerebral dysfunction covering a wide range of signs and symptoms has been widely adopted (Francis-Williams 1963, Graham and Rutter 1968, Köng 1963, Knobloch and Pasamanick 1959, Paine 1966, Paine *et al.* 1968, Stevens *et al.* 1967, Stutte 1966, Werry 1968, Wigglesworth 1961, 1963). However, the validity of this concept has been queried (Birch *et al.* 1964, Gomez 1967, Ingram 1963, 1966, Mac Keith 1963, McFie 1963, Pond 1960, Work and Haldane 1966). The diversity of opinion in these various studies testifies to the extremely complex nature of the relationship between brain functions and overt behaviour.

In classical neurology there was a strong belief in the mapping of brain functions. It is true that, in the adult organism, certain circumscribed lesions in specific parts of the brain are consistently accompanied by specific behavioural aberrations. For example, parietal lobe lesions lead to a disorder of the timing and sequence of voluntary motor behaviour (apraxia) and a number of cognitive dysfunctions, limbic lesions lead to emotional disturbances, and cerebellar lesions lead to instability of goal-directed motor activity (*e.g.* voluntary reaching and grasping).

New techniques are now available to the clinician in his search for structural alteration or functional abnormality in a particular region of the brain which might account for a specific behavioural phenomenon. These include pneumo-, echo- and electroencephalography, arteriography and scintillography. It is now evident that a simple direct relationship between brain lesion and alteration in behaviour is less common than has been previously supposed. Symptoms may occur only temporarily, such as focal irritation in temporal lobe epilepsy. Apart from the ictal phenomenon, behaviour may remain relatively uninfluenced even when a dysfunction of a part of the brain cannot be denied. Slowly developing processes may destroy large areas of the brain before any symptoms are evident. In other cases, behavioural phenomena cannot be related to lesions in specific brain regions, though they may be considered 'organic' in origin (*e.g.* organic psychoses on toxic or other bases).

The relationship between brain and behaviour is different in the developing infantile brain. It is known that comparable brain lesions in infant and adult animals differ in their behavioural sequelae, from experiments with monkeys (Kling and Tucker 1968, Thompson *et al.* 1969, Tucker and Kling 1969), with cats (Benjamin and Thompson 1959, Kling 1965, Scharlock *et al.* 1963, Wetzel *et al.* 1965) and with rats (Kling 1966, Schwartz and Kling 1964). There is no reason to assume that this does not also apply in man. Thus, our knowledge of particular behaviour sequelae of specific localised lesions in adults is not applicable to children.

Very often, however, the lesion is not localised, but there are diffuse changes to the nervous system consisting of scattered cell-damage and cell-loss and patchy destruction of myelin sheaths. This may be due to pre- or perinatal anoxia (anoxic anoxia) or circulatory failure (stagnant anoxia). The pattern of damage to the brain depends on the developmental stage of the nervous system.

Early intra-uterine malnutrition, which interferes with the DNA synthesis and proliferation processes in the nervous system (Dobbing 1968, Osofsky 1969, Winick 1969) may be another source of diffuse damage. In rats, it may lead to an under-development of 10-25 per cent of the brain weight, and similar effects are now reported in infants. The effects of the insulted brain development on behaviour, however, are still widely unknown.

Despite a volume of work on these subjects, surprisingly few papers discuss in detail the neurological examination which will identify children with neurological dysfunction. Reliable assessments of behavioural problems have been made by psychologists for many years; similarly standardized techniques of neurological examination are urgently required. This is particularly true with regard to children whose signs of brain dysfunction are not gross and obvious to the clinician, but occur in rather inconspicuous form. Even recent publications on the neurological examination in infancy and childhood (Müller 1968, Paine and Oppé 1966) pay little attention to the problems of diagnosis arising in such cases. This book may therefore fulfil a worthwhile function in providing a description of the neurological examination procedure for the detection of minor nervous dysfunction in children as developed in our department.

CHAPTER 1

The Design of a Neurological Examination Technique for the Detection of Minor Neurological Signs

A neurological examination should be a comprehensive assessment of neural functions and should therefore be as complete as possible. It must also be reliable in the sense of being replicable by the same and different examiners, and it should be based on objective criteria.

Neurological examinations of children have been carried out by many examiners and this has resulted in variations in the design of the technique according to personal preferences and tastes. It would be impossible to construct a method which would incorporate all the many tests that have been described. A compromise is inevitable. The reasons for our selection of tests are outlined below.

The least problematic aspect of the neurological examination is the assessment of a large variety of motor functions which, observed in standardized conditions, can be objectively described and quantified. This category comprises posture, spontaneous movements, resistance against passive movements, muscle power, reflexes and locomotion.

Sensory functions which relate to movement can also be easily assessed. These include oculo-motor and pupillary responses, nystagmus, gross pain (withdrawal responses) and proprioceptors (muscle spindles).

However, all those sensory qualities in which perception can only be assessed by verbal report or by imitation are subject to erroneous interpretation, because of their dependance on the language development and mental capacity of the patient. Thus, it is extremely difficult to obtain reliable data about light touch or differences in pain perception in children, particularly children with behavioural problems and/or mental deficiency. The examiner will obtain nothing more than vague and subjective impressions. Similar pitfalls hamper the assessment of two-point discrimination and stereognosis, in which the intelligence and motivation of the child play an important role.

Clearly, the examiner must be aware that an investigation of one function necessarily involves the use of others. This is important when a child does not pass a test. If he wishes to give an unequivocal interpretation of the finding, the examiner must ascertain the cause of the child's failure; this is often extremely difficult. For example, in a test of visual acuity such as the Snellen Letter Charts, the Sheridan-Gardner tests or even picture charts, the child's success indicates that visual acuity has been tested. However, in the case of failure the examiner must remember that the test investigates not only visual acuity but also the child's ability to recognise objects and to verbalize. Failure does not necessarily imply impaired visual acuity, particularly in the case of children with behavioural difficulties who may show short attention span and poor concentration. These factors may considerably affect the child's ultimate score, and it would therefore be preferable to refer such children to an ophthalmologist, who can often obtain better and more objective data about visual acuity by skiascopy.

A distinction should be made between deviant findings which are interpretable in terms of neural mechanisms and those which are multiply determined, because learning, social conditions and innumerable other environmental factors influence the performance. The result of a tap on the patellar tendon can be easily related to particular neural mechanisms. Visual acuity, however, is multi-conditioned.

The same can be said of many tests used in the assessment of motor coordination. If a child is asked to pick up matches and put them in a match-box, the examiner may get an impression of his ability to manipulate small objects. The quantification of the performance per time unit in terms of the number of matches placed accurately in the box (most of the items in the Oseretsky battery are of this type) does not make it an unequivocal neurological test, because of the multi-interpretability of the result. In addition to motor coordination, many other factors are involved, such as visuo-motor abilities, general intelligence, motivation, attention span, etc.

An analogous reasoning is valid for the 'imitation of gestures' test (Bergès and Lézine 1965).

In designing a specific technique for the neurological examination, it is clearly necessary to obviate complex behavioural data masquerading as neurological items. For instance, if an unspecific hyperkinesis is evaluated as an abnormal neurological *symptom*, despite our lack of knowledge about its organic basis, this type of behavioural difficulty will automatically be interpreted as a neurological *sign*. Fluctuating attention or a short attention span, whether observed or reported in the history, cannot be taken as evidence of brain dysfunction *per se*. If a child has neurological signs which clearly indicate brain dysfunction, one may conclude that there may be an organic basis for the behavioural problems. However, definite proof will still be missing.

In our selection of tests, we have tried to look at as many parameters of neuro-logical function as possible, and to use more than one test within each parameter. In some instances it would be possible to extend the number of tests used. For example, many more reflexes than are described here could easily be incorporated. However, we feel that an increase in the number of reflexes tested in a routine examination does not correspondingly increase the amount of information obtained, and we excluded them for practical reasons.

With regard to sensory function, we found that many of the classical tests of adult neurology were not sensitive enough to detect disturbances in children with relatively minor dysfunction. In children with more severe neurological disorder, *e.g.* a hemiplegic, it may be possible to use the classical tests of sensory function to identify a gross sensory loss such as the loss of light touch all over the hemiplegic limb. Even in these circumstances, however, an assessment will only be reliable if the child is old enough and sufficiently intelligent and well-motivated to reply to the examiner's questions. In children with behavioural difficulties, too, we found it very difficult to account for the findings with, for example, two-point discrimination, even in nine- to ten-year-old children. The responses obtained were inconsistent and unreliable from one examination to the next. We feel, therefore, that such tests are not worth carrying out in these children as a routine. In individual cases, it may be useful to carry out a separate, extensive examination of sensory functions.

The child's speech and language deserve special comment. This aspect of behaviour is clearly of particular interest to the developmental neurologist and to all doctors who deal with children. Some types of speech disorders can be specifically related to brain damage, as is well known from adult neurology. Delayed and abnormal speech development in children may arouse a strong suspicion of neurological damage. However, it is difficult to be certain that neurological damage is the cause of their abnormality. An accurate assessment of speech and language requires a skilled technique. In our opinion, such a description is a task for someone with special experience in assessing this particular function and should not be included within the general neurological examination. It is often possible to get a general impression of the child's speech during the course of the examination and to refer the child for a separate, detailed examination of this function, if this is judged desirable.

One final point must be considered. A distinction is often made between 'soft' and 'hard' neurological signs, the import of which is open to serious doubt. One cannot escape the impression that this dichotomy is based on soft and hard methods and/or interpretation, rather than soft and hard abnormalities of brain function. Pseudo-diagnostic terms such as 'hard' and 'soft' should be omitted.*

ESSENTIAL CONSIDERATIONS

Developmental Approach

The nervous system of an infant or child is in a phase of rapid development and therefore the examiner's approach must be age-specific. It is essential for him to be familiar with the maturational processes of motor patterns and sensory mechanisms. Our technique is adapted to the maturation of the nervous system from its early stages of relatively low organisation to the increasing organisation of later stages. This type of examination is based on concepts and techniques fundamentally different from those applied in pediatric neurology which have been extrapolated from adult neurology.

In addition, great caution should be exercised if neuro-physiological data derived from animal experiments are applied as analoguous. For example, an analysis of patterns of spasticity in the cat should not be used as an explanation of the patterns seen in a child. There is evidence of gross differences of nervous functioning between species, and erroneous conclusions may easily be drawn if infantile brain mechanisms are interpreted on the basis of animal studies (Prechtl and Lenard 1968).

Behavioural State

The behavioural state of the child is an important variable which greatly influences the results of the examination. With regard to the young infant, an accurate evaluation of the behavioural state during the examination is essential for an interpretation of the findings (Prechtl and Beintema 1964). For example, an increased resistance to passive movements found in a vigorously moving, crying infant may mean something quite different from the same finding in a quiet or even sleeping infant. Similarly,

*After completion of this manuscript, Rutter and co-workers (1970) published their Isle of Wight study, in which they discuss extensively several of the points dealt with in the introduction and in this paragraph.

TABLE I
Behavioural state

0*	= awake, not crying
1	= awake, fussing
2	= awake, crying**
3	= yelling**
4	= other (describe)

Scale starts with '0' for reasons of coding on punch cards.
**If crying or yelling persists for any length of time, the examination procedure must be discontinued.*

the behavioural state of preschool and school-age children must also be taken into account. Clearly, the examination is only possible if the child is awake and therefore his behavioural state need only be recorded in terms of the degree of disturbance. (The scale for the behavioural state is given in Table I.) If the child's disturbed behaviour persists, the examiner must attempt to pacify him. Should he fail to do so, the examination may have to be discontinued. The child's state must be recorded on the proforma (see page 93) at the beginning of each section of the examination. Changes of state during the course of one section can be recorded in a special column on the right side of the proforma.

In contrast to the examination of the young infant, there is a second aspect of the behavioural state which plays an important role in the assessment of children: the co-operativeness of the child may determine the validity of the findings. Obviously, this will relate to his behavioural state as described above. Co-operation is expressed in terms of social responsiveness, *i.e.* the way in which the child responds to the examiner's handling and instructions. In this context the scoring is mainly concerned with the validity of the neurological findings and not with a psychiatric appraisal of the child's behaviour. It is sufficient to cover the range of manifestations from positive to negative, using unequivocal descriptions of behaviour that might influence test results, without making any inferences about the underlying mechanisms of that behaviour. The scale for social responsiveness is given in Table II and must be routinely recorded at the end of each section of the examination. Changes in social responsiveness during the course of a section can be noted in a special column on the right side of the proforma opposite the relevant items.

TABLE II
Social responsiveness

0*	= interested, agrees with proposals, no stimulation needed, facial expression alert.
1	= disinterested, but agrees with proposals, no particular encouragement needed, but not facially alert.
2	= reluctant, needs encouragement, appears anxious, tense facial expression.
3	= reluctant, needs encouragement, appears sullen, withdrawn.
4	= shrinks back on approach, refuses to fulfill demands, appears frightened.
5	= refuses to fulfill demands, appears impassive.
6	= resists by pushing examiner away, tries to get away, struggles.
7	= other (describe).

Scale starts with '0' for reasons of coding on punch cards.

It is, of course, important to keep the child as co-operative as possible during the examination. Tests which are least likely to disturb him are carried out first, and all procedures which might excite or frighten him are postponed to the end. This technique results in a sequence of tests which is in no way logical in terms of brain topography or of functional systems, as is usual in adult neurology, but which does help to avoid many difficulties.

As the child's behavioural state may be influenced by fatigue, the time at which the examination is carried out must be recorded. It is also necessary to obtain adequate information about factors such as drugs taken by the child and the time of his last meal, as these may influence not only his behavioural state but also the results of the tests.

Environmental Conditions and Technique of Handling the Patient

The behavioural state of the child is strongly influenced by environmental conditions and these need to be standardized. Certain aspects of special importance are discussed here, as some doctors tend to consider them minor points and disregard them. This may account for difficulties in obtaining reliable results. We ourselves have never found any difficulty in carrying out a funduscopic examination, for example, since by the end of the session the child is relaxed and co-operative.

Undressing*

In general, children dislike being undressed during the examination. Young children get particularly tense and this may impede a reliable assessment. This difficulty will diminish in the case of older children over the age of seven, although boys are often extremely bashful and tense during the examination of the cremasteric reflex.

To alleviate these problems, undressing should be adapted to the needs of the examination. The child does not need to remain undressed the whole time, and in our experience it is preferable that he should stay undressed for as short a time as possible. However, he should take off his shoes and socks at the beginning of the examination and remain barefoot throughout, otherwise accurate observation of posture and motility of the feet and legs is not possible. Muscle power and resistance to passive movements can be tested before the child needs to remove any more clothing; for the testing of tendon reflexes, he must remove outer clothing so that his arms and legs are bare; and the examination of the trunk requires further undressing. Obviously undressing in stages will often take up a lot of time, but this is compensated for by the child's improved social responsiveness and loss of tension.

It is often advisable for the examiner, rather than the mother or nurse, to help the child get dressed again, as many children find this reassuring. Once the child is dressed and convinced of the friendly nature of the examination, the assessment of the head (funduscopy, testing of the corneal and gag reflexes and inspection of the pharyngeal arches), which often frightens young children, can be carried out with relative ease.

*In order to demonstrate the procedures and responses more clearly, the children appearing in the illustrations in this book were undressed for the examination.

The Examination Couch

Many children, particularly those aged below six, are frightened by examination couches which are usually too high, narrow and cold. As a result, they are unable to relax, thus impeding the course of the examination. However, most items of the neurological examination can be tested while the child is sitting or standing. If a couch is absolutely essential, it should be reasonably low and broad, and covered with a soft mattress. A mat on the floor often provides the best means of carrying out parts of the examination when the child has to lie down (*e.g.* the knee-heel test, testing of the hip-joints, inspection of the spine and the posture of the legs in prone and supine position). The abdominal skin, Galant and cremasteric reflexes are elicitable, when present, in the standing child. It is also easier to examine muscle power, resistance against passive movements (in most joints) and reflexes, which require a relaxed subject, when the child is sitting rather than lying down. For this purpose, an ordinary wooden chair without arms can generally be used. The child's feet must not touch the floor, so older children may have to sit on the edge of the table; a music-stool of adjustable height may also be used, provided its surface is not round and convex, since this would influence the child's sitting posture. Certain specific tests, such as tests for dyskinesia and diadochokinesis, are best done when the child is standing.

The Examination Room

Clearly, the room where the examination takes place should be quiet and restful as regards sight and sound, so that the child may feel at ease. A doctor's examination room often contains an amount of frightening paraphernalia, which should be avoided, as should the examiner's white coat which children, particularly those with repeated experience of medical care, find frightening. In addition, the room, and the examiner's hands too, should be pleasantly warm.

The Presence of the Mother

The advisability of allowing a parent of other familiar adult to be present during the examination has been much disputed, and often depends more on the examiner than on the child. General rules cannot be given but, for the examination of groups with an aim to statistical analysis, it is advisable to keep the environmental situation the same in all cases. We would therefore suggest that mothers of children up to the age of six should be asked to be present, while older children should be seen alone.

Relationship with the Child

The initial moments of the interview often determine the course of the examination, and we have found that it is important not to approach the child directly at the beginning. An introductory talk to the mother while the child is listening and playing with a toy placed near him by the examiner will often impress the child more than a direct explanation. After a few minutes the examiner may make a direct remark to the child who has had time to familiarize himself with his surroundings. An adequate period of adaptation should be allowed and it might be worthwhile noting its duration.

During this period, the examiner can observe posture and motility, which may give clues to be followed up at a later phase of the examination.

It is important that the examination procedure should be playful wherever possible (in the examination of muscle power, for instance) so as to reassure the child. The order of the examination was designed with this in mind.

Another point that the examiner should consider is that he is likely to tower above the sitting and even the standing child. He should therefore avoid standing up or leaning over the child, but sit or squat beside or opposite him. When he has to move around, he should do so as inconspicuously as possible.

THE COURSE OF THE EXAMINATION

The examination consists of:

(1) an observation of the child's motor behaviour, and

(2) testing of specific nervous functions.

In general the examiner should keep to the course of the examination as set out in this book. The procedure is divided into several sections. All the items which can be assessed while the child is sitting down are carried out first, followed by an examination while the child is standing. Locomotion is then tested. An assessment in the lying position is left almost to the end of the procedure, and is followed by the last section, namely, the examination of the head.

At the beginning and end of each section, the child's behavioural state and degree of social responsiveness are always recorded. During a section, a subsequent recording may be necessary if a change occurs or if specific tests require an extra assessment, as in the case of the test for dyskinesia. The examiner should allow himself some degree of flexibility within each section and remember that his main aim is to ensure that the child is not disturbed by the examination and remains as responsive as possible.

This method is specifically designed for the detection of minor neurological dysfunction, and most emphasis in the discussion of the findings is placed on their meaning in relation to this. However, brief mention must be made of their significance in relation to more serious conditions, as minor signs may be the first manifestations of a progressive illness. Single abnormal signs are rarely of much significance in isolation; a comprehensive examination is necessary to evaluate the child's neurological status. One should always approach the interpretation of single tests with care, but for practical reasons the possible significance of each test is mentioned after a description of the procedure and recording.

Each test item of the proforma in each section is discussed separately, and in each case relevant age variables are mentioned, the technique of eliciting a response is described (*i.e.* the position of the child and the examiner, the method of procedure and the response itself), the way of recording the response is indicated and some remarks are made about the significance of the response and its relationship to the child's age. These remarks do not pretend to give a complete outline of the significance or a differential diagnosis of all responses. As stated previously, this book is primarily a methodological and not a clinical textbook.

The responses are measured numerically: the absence of a response is always scored as 0, a weak response as 1, a clear response as 2, a strong response as 3, etc.

This must be taken into account in the final interpretation. In the case of responses which are normally *present*, the optimal score will usually be 2; a weak response which may be non-optimal scores 1; a strong response which may also be non-optimal scores 3 or 4. This applies to tendon reflexes and resistance against passive movements, for example. However, in the case of the plantar grasp response, which should be *absent*, the optimal score will be 0, while scores of 1 or 2 reflect non-optimal responses, *i.e.* the presence of the response.

After the description of the full examination, the interrelation of signs and their cohesion into syndromes is discussed, followed by a critical annotation of their possible relationship to behaviour. It must be stressed again that a single neurological sign very rarely has any clinical significance. Only the number and possible inter-relationship of signs can give a guide to the interpretation of results. On completion of the examination, the examiner collates the abnormal signs recorded descriptively during the examination, and attempts to see how they hang together and whether they form a recognised syndrome. Quite often he will find a number of unrelated signs and no clearcut syndrome, so that it may perhaps be possible to speak of a syndrome consisting of the absence of a syndrome.

CHAPTER 2

Assessment of the Child Sitting

General Remarks

As indicated previously, the behavioural state of the child (Table I) should be recorded at the beginning of the examination and at the beginning of each set of tests. Social responsiveness (Table II) should be recorded at the end of each set of tests. Any change in either state or responsiveness during the course of a section should be noted in the appropriate column. It is also worthwhile recording both aspects before and after the child takes off his shoes and socks.

Behavioural State

The optimal state of the child for the following series of tests is 0, though the tests may be continued if the behavioural state is 1.

Position

The child is asked to sit up straight on a chair without supporting himself with his arms or elbows. The chair should preferably be a simple upright one with no arms. The child's feet should not touch the floor and older children may be asked to sit on a table. If the child's posture seems abnormal, it may be advisable to ask him to get up and walk around before sitting down again.

When the child is sitting down, it is very important to see that the head is kept in the midline and that the posture of the body and limbs is symmetrical. A slight tendency towards an asymmetric tonic neck response pattern, for instance, may be present and influence findings. If a child cannot centre his head or keep it centred, this must be recorded. In the case of torticollis, passive centring of the head means a change of tension in the neck muscles on both sides, and this can influence the findings on other tests. Postural deviations of the body may have similar results.

Posture

Age

This test is suitable for children aged 5 to 10, but is difficult to assess in children below the age of 5.

Procedure

The examiner inspects the posture of the head, body and legs. He should pay special attention to any tilting or rotation of the head and rotation or bending, either forward or backward, of the spine. A slight scoliosis may go unobserved as the child is at this point barefoot but otherwise fully dressed.

Recording

Any persistent deviations from a symmetrical upright posture are described by noting the appropriate score in the relevant place on the proforma. Posture of the head, trunk, legs and feet is scored for the following aspects.

Head:	rotated		
	bent laterally		
	ante- and retroflexion		
Trunk:	rotated		
	bent laterally		
	kyphosis		
	lordosis		
	symmetrically collapsed		
Legs:	endorotation	flexion	abduction
	exorotation	extension	adduction
Feet:	endorotation	dorsiflexion	abduction
	exorotation	plantar flexion	adduction

The scores range from 0 to 2, 0 indicating that the description is not valid, 2 that the description is manifestly valid. Each side of the body is scored separately on the corresponding side of the proforma, unless otherwise indicated. If, for instance, a child sits with one knee slightly more flexed than the other, and this is a consistent finding, the score for the more flexed side would be 1 (often in that instance there will be a slightly increased adduction of the same leg). This does not necessarily indicate an abnormality, but merely records a difference between the two sides.

Significance

In all cases, the optimal score is 0, indicating a neutral posture. Sometimes a child may have slightly bent shoulders, which he can hold straight on request, but which droop again after a moment; as a rule this is not pathological. A final conclusion can only be reached when the examination of posture while standing and during movement has been completed and the sensorimotor apparatus has been adequately tested. When a child is sitting, it is quite normal for some degree of lordosis or kyphosis to be present; lordosis may be particularly prominent in slender girls.

A consistently maintained asymmetrical posture should always arouse a suspicion of pathology which will be confirmed or dispelled during the rest of the examination. Deviations due to obvious bone or muscle deformities need not be mentioned here. A slightly abnormal posture may result from muscular weakness on one or both sides of the body. Lateral incurvations of the trunk may indicate a scoliosis, and this must be checked when the child is standing and lying down. If present, there may be a skeletal anomaly.

Lateral turning of the head may be due to visual difficulties, *e.g.* suppression of diplopia, originating from paresis of the musculus rectus lateralis of one eye, or compensation for a homonymous hemianopia.

An asymmetrical posture of the freely hanging legs, often most clearly indicated by the position of the feet, may originate from or be one of the first manifestations of a hemisyndrome (see page 84). On the other hand, static causes, originating in the hip-joint, the ankle or the foot, must also be borne in mind.

Spontaneous Motility

Age

    This test is suitable for all children aged 3 to 10.

Procedure

    An observation of spontaneous motility can be carried out initially during the introductory talk to the mother when the child is sitting and playing with a toy. Quantity and quality of movement must be taken into account, and a distinction made between gross and small movements in each instance.

    In *gross movements*, body and limbs all participate. The child may arch his back, turn round in the chair, swing his legs, etc. Eventually, gross movements will result in spatial displacements, the child jumping off the chair, walking round the room, climbing over the furniture, opening the door, etc.

    In *small movements*, only parts of the body or limbs are involved. The child may be restless and fidget with hands or fingers, make faces, wiggle his toes or fidget with buttons, clothes or other objects, but his position changes relatively little, if at all.

    The quantity and quality of the movements are estimated as indicated below, and special attention must be paid to the occurrence of involuntary movements such as tremor, choreiform movements or slight dystonic movements (see page 36).

Recording

(a) *Quantity*

Gross movements:

    0 = no movements. The child sits perfectly still for at least 3 minutes.

    1 = a few movements only. The child stays on the chair, but turns round a bit, swings his legs, etc.

    2 = a moderate amount of movements. The child stays on the chair, but turns round repeatedly, arches his back, swings his legs, etc.

    3 = an excessive amount of movements. The child is continuously on the move, jumps on and off the chair, wanders round the room, etc.

Small movements:

    0 = no movements. The child sits perfectly still for at least 3 minutes.

    1 = a few movements only, mainly of hands and face.

    2 = a moderate amount of movements. The child moves his hands and feet, but not continuously.

    3 = an excessive amount of movements. The child fidgets continuously, cannot keep his hands or feet still, plucks at his clothing, etc.

11

(*b*) *Quality*

Speed: 0 = the child sits perfectly still.
1 = the movements are performed slowly.
2 = the movements are performed at a moderate tempo.
3 = all movements are performed very rapidly.

Smoothness: 0 = the child sits perfectly still.
1 = all movements are very smooth and supple.
2 = movements are mostly smooth and supple, often depending on their speed.
3 = movements are performed clumsily and may be abrupt and jerky, often giving the impression of being broken down into constituent parts.
4 = all movements are performed very awkwardly or are very abrupt and jerky.

Adequacy: 0 = the child sits perfectly still.
1 = movements are easily goal-directed.
2 = some movements are goal-directed, others are inadequate and do not serve a clear purpose.
3 = the child moves around aimlessly; his movements are mainly inadequate.

(*c*) *Involuntary movements*

Type and localisation are described if present (see page 36).

Significance

A score of 3 for quantity of gross movements denotes overactivity, a score of 3 for quantity of small movements denotes a restless or fidgety child. However, these descriptions do not indicate a diagnosis of 'hyperkinesis' which is the descriptive term for a behavioural category. It is necessary to record the quantity of spontaneous motility, but it is the quality of movement which is truly significant for an understanding of the child's neurological functioning.

Speed, smoothness and adequacy may not be equally affected; high scores for speed are not always paralleled by high scores for smoothness and adequacy. In some overactive children, all aspects may be scored highly, denoting a rapidly moving child whose movements are jerky and abrupt and often inadequate. Children with awkward and clumsy motility will often show low scores for quantity and speed of movements. Younger children (aged below six) will normally show more movements than older children.

Evidently, if involuntary movements such as choreiform movements or tremor are present, smoothness will be affected, but quantity, speed and adequacy of isolated movements may well be within the normal range.

Once more, it must be stressed that single observations are not a sufficient basis for conclusions which can only be reached after a complete examination. Spontaneous motility is observed again when the child is standing at a later stage in the procedure.

Kicking

Age

This test is suitable for children aged 3 to 6, and for older children who fail the knee-heel test (see page 64).

Procedure

The examiner holds out his hand on a level with the child's knee at such a distance that the child can easily touch it with his foot. The child is asked to touch the examiner's palm with his toes. The test is carried out with the hand in three positions for each foot; first the examiner holds out his hand directly in front of the child and the child is asked to kick three times; then he holds out his hand at a 45° angle to the left and then to the right of the child for three kicks each time.

Response

The child kicks the examiner's hand, scoring a point for each hit. The highest score for each leg is thus 9.

Recording

The number of kicks for each leg is recorded quantitatively in each position, so that the total score can be quickly calculated.

Significance

This is mainly a test of the co-ordination of the legs for children who cannot or will not do the knee-heel test. A discrepancy between right and left may be related to dominance, and an interpretation is only possible in combination with findings from the rest of the examination. Performance is correlated with age; the child can normally perform perfectly with both legs by the age of six.

ASSESSMENT OF THE MOTOR SYSTEM

Age

These tests are suitable for all children aged 3 to 10.

General Remarks

The assessment is divided into three aspects: active power, resistance against passive movements and range of movements. The neck, shoulders, elbows, wrists, knees and ankles are tested separately for all three categories. Examination of the hip-joint is postponed until the end of the examination when the child is lying on the examination table.

French authors such as André-Thomas *et al.* (1960) and Tardieu (1968) have made valuable contributions to the study of tone and many tests have been described for use in such an assessment. We feel that many of these tests are difficult to standardize, and that as much information can be gained from the use of much simpler tests.

13

Muscle Power

Procedure

The child is asked to grasp the examiner's fingers as tightly as possible, using both hands at the same time. The examiner must resist voluntary flexion and extension of the elbow. Abduction and adduction of the arm against resistance provides an estimation of the power of the arm and shoulder muscles.

Pronation and supination should be carefully tested as, in its early stages, a paresis may manifest itself in the muscles used for these movements (*e.g.* in muscular dystrophy). The examiner must take hold of the child's hand as if to shake hands and ask him to pronate and supinate against resistance.

The strength of the hip and thigh muscles is examined at the end of the procedure when the child is lying on the examination table (for flexion, extension, abduction and adduction). Flexion and extension of the knee joint and the strength of the ankle and foot movements can be tested while the child is sitting.

After testing for power of movement against resistance, the child is asked to keep various joints still while the examiner tries to move them.

Recording

The muscle power tested in these two ways is recorded as a compound score for each joint (see proforma). We feel that the well known Medical Research Council scale is not really useful in the case of children with minor dysfunction of the nervous system, since such children are unlikely to exhibit muscular weakness so severe that they are unable to make movements against gravity. Several ratings of the MRC scale have therefore been omitted, but approximate equivalents to our own scale are given in brackets.

      0 = no active movements (MRC 0, 1, 2, and partially 3).

      1 = active movements present, but unable to overcome more than slight resistance (MRC partially 3, and 4).

      2 = active movements present, and able to counteract moderately strong resistance (MRC 5).

      3 = active movements present, and able to overcome very strong resistance (MRC partially 5).

Resistance against Passive Movements (Figs 1-6)

Procedure

The child is asked to relax as much as possible and resistance is tested and assessed by passively moving the various joints.

The examiner first takes the child's head in his hands and gently bends it forward, backward and to each side. The shoulder joint is tested by holding the shoulder girdle firm with one hand and moving the child's upper arm through the range of movements of the shoulder joint with the other. To test the elbow, the upper arm is held firm while the lower arm is flexed and extended; to test the wrist joint, the lower arm is held firm in a semiflexed position (to avoid pronation and supination which is tested separately) and the hand is moved.

While the child is sitting, the position of the hip-joint can be standardized by

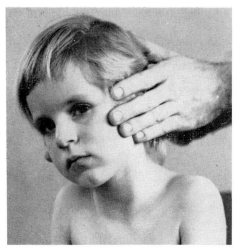 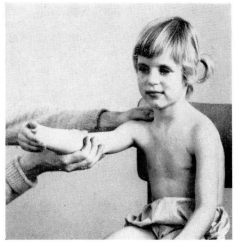

Fig. 1. Examination of resistance to passive movements in the neck. The head is gently moved to the side.

Fig. 2. Examination of resistance to passive movements in the right shoulder.

holding the upper leg firm, so that the resistance of the knee can be tested. To test the ankle joint, the lower leg is held firm with the knee in a semiflexed position.

The passive movements must be carried out slowly and carefully, and should be repeated several times.

Recording

Resistance against passive movements is recorded as a compound score for each joint (see proforma, page 93).

0 = complete lack of resistance
1 = weak resistance
2 = moderately strong resistance
3 = strong resistance

Range of Passive Movements
Procedure

In testing resistance to passive movements, the joints are moved through their full range, and hyperextensibility or limitation of movements is recorded. The range of movements shows wide individual variation. The average range of movements for the various joints is as follows:

(*a*) *Head*	Anteflexion:	the chin can touch the chest.
	Retroflexion:	an imaginary plane from mentum to occiput approaches the horizontal.
	Rotation:	180° from side to side.
(*b*) *Shoulder*	Abduction:	to ± 110° with shoulder girdle held firm.
	Anteflexion:	to ± 100° with shoulder girdle held firm.

15

		Retroflexion:	to $\pm$ 60° with shoulder girdle held firm.

Retroflexion: to $\pm$ 60° with shoulder girdle held firm.
Other movements are not considered.

(c)	Elbow	Extension:	to 180°.
		Flexion:	to $\pm$ 20°, depending on the thickness of the arm.
(d)	Wrist	Extension:	to 70° with lower arm.
		Flexion:	to 90° with lower arm.
(e)	Knees	Extension:	to 180°.
		Flexion:	depending on the bulk of the leg.
(f)	Ankles	The range of movement from dorsiflexion to plantarflexion is 100°/110°.	

Recording

Only the degree of deviation from the average range of movements mentioned above is recorded, and should be quantified as far as possible, for instance, by using a goniometer (Holt 1965).

Significance

Decreased active power may result from neuromuscular disease (see below), paresis or general weakness as an unspecific symptom of a number of disorders, such as infectious diseases, metabolic disturbances or malnutrition. A slight decrease may be the first manifestation of a progressive disorder; cases of unilateral decrease in muscle strength should be noted with particular care.

A thorough discussion of the causes of increased and decreased resistance against passive movements is beyond the scope of this book, which is principally concerned with minor, often inconspicuous, deviations from optimal functioning. Nevertheless, the examiner must bear in mind that in extreme cases, a slight alteration in resistance to passive movements may be one of the first signs of a progressive disorder of the neuromuscular system (*e.g.* leuco-dystrophies, cerebro-retinal degenerations, dyskinesias such as Huntington's chorea, cerebral neoplasms or toxic degenerations such as lead poisoning).

Table III provides a review of the main causes of neuromuscular weakness in

TABLE III
Causes of neuromuscular weakness in childhood

(a) Unspecific: infectious diseases metabolic disorders malnutrition convalescence from serious illness	(c) Neuropathies (d) Disorders of the neuromuscular junction: myasthenia gravis
(b) Disorders of the C.N.S.: perinatal C.N.S. damage leucodystrophies metabolic disorders myelopathies	(e) Myopathies: muscular dystrophies (dermato) myositis congenital non-progressive myopathies myotonic syndromes periodic paralysis

N.B. Adapted from Munsat and Pearson 1967.

16

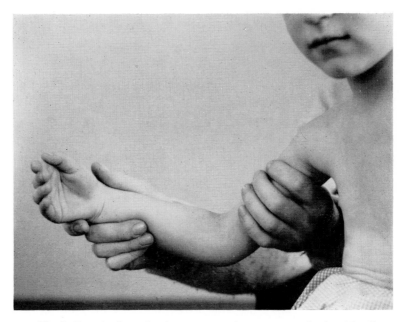

Fig. 3. Examination of resistance to passive movements in the right elbow.

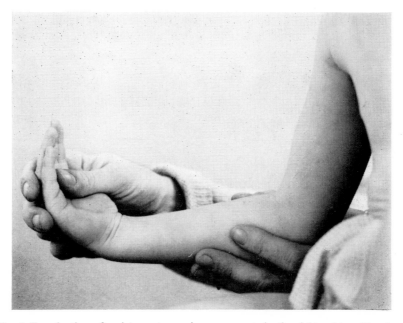

Fig. 4. Examination of resistance to passive movements in the right wrist and hand.

17

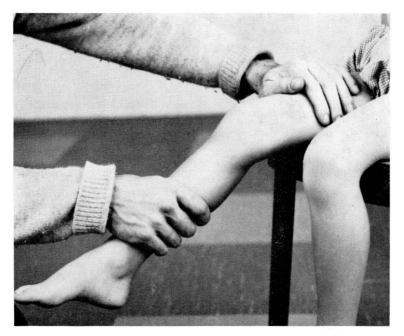

Fig. 5. Examination of resistance to passive movements in the right knee.

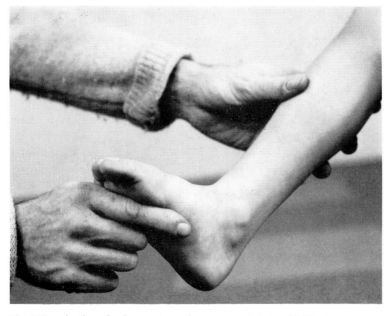

Fig. 6. Examination of resistance to passive movements in the right foot.

childhood. It should be noted that disturbances of the afferent input to the spinal cord (afferent nerves, spinal ganglion, dorsal roots or dorsal columns) may result in a decreased resistance to passive movements before other signs are present. In cases of hypotonia, not all muscles are necessarily involved at the same time. One may be impaired while others function normally, *e.g.* the peroneal muscle of the lower leg (see test for walking on heels, page 54).

Often a decreased resistance against passive movements is found in mentally retarded children. Children who turn out to be spastic at the age of two to three years may also show a decreased resistance against passive movements during early infancy. On the other hand, a slight decrease of resistance to passive movements may be found in young preschool children and disappear in the course of the years.

It is also beyond the scope of this book to discuss the differentiation between spasticity, 'lead-pipe' rigidity and 'cog-wheel' rigidity, since these phenomena evidently surpass the bounds of minor nervous dysfunction. An increased resistance to passive movements, if not of central nervous system origin, may be due to myogenic (scleroderma, acute myositis) or articular (acute or chronic rheumatoid arthritis) disorders. Conclusions as to origin and diagnosis in an individual patient can only be made when the examination has been completed.

Particularly in five- to eight-year-old children, a slight but consistent discrepancy can sometimes be found between the resistance against passive movements in the left and right limbs. Often there seems to exist a relationship with handedness and footedness, which at this stage of the examination has not been assessed. Usually the dominant arm and leg show greater resistance. It may be that the discrepancy is the result of a differential development of the muscle-bulk on the dominant side. It is also possible, however, that the complete assessment may reveal signs that constitute a definite pattern with which such a discrepancy is congruent, indicating the presence of a hemisyndrome (see page 84).

The range of movements of the joints may vary considerably from child to child, especially with regard to the degree of extension. Slenderly built girls have wider ranges of movements than more heavily built boys of the same age. Children aged three to four may have a slightly smaller range of movements than children aged four and over, whose muscular system is better developed. A classic case is the three-year-old with a rather protruberant belly and slightly rounded shoulders, who often shows a slightly decreased range of movements of the joints. However, between the ages of three and seven, flexibility of the joints is not related to age; variations commonly occur not only between children but also between the various joints of the individual child.

An abnormal increase in the range of movements is generally related to a low resistance against passive movements. Limitation of movements may originate in the ligaments of the joints, the muscles or the motor neurone. Complaints of pain during the examination should be very carefully investigated. Testing the range of movements may be painful, particularly where there are articular or myogenic limitations of movement, and this pain may in turn cause further limitation of movement during the examination. Spontaneous pain caused by acute arthritis or dermomyositis,

19

for example, or even from any other origin, may decrease the range of movements by causing an inability to relax the musculature, thus interfering with the optimal range of movements basically present. Persistent asymmetries should always be carefully considered, since they may be part of a hemisyndrome. This conclusion can only be drawn on completion of the entire examination, when other causes (*e.g.* local or peripheral) can be excluded.

CHAPTER 3

Examination of Reflexes

General Remarks

During the examination of the reflexes (including the plantar reflex, the abdominal skin reflex and the cremasteric reflex which are tested at a later stage), the examiner should bear in mind that the responses may diminish after one or two trials. If several trials are required for the same reflex, there should be an interval of sometimes even a few minutes between each trial.

Behavioural State

The optimal state of the child for the following tests is 0, though the assessment can proceed if it is 1.

Position

The child may remain sitting on either table or chair. During the elicitation of reflexes, the posture of the arms and legs should be symmetrical and the child's head should be centred in the midline.

Age

These tests are suitable for all children aged 3 to 10.

Ankle Jerk (Fig. 7)

Procedure

We have found that most children are more relaxed sitting down than lying on an examination table or kneeling on a chair. It is important that the feet should hang freely and that the muscles of the knee and ankle joints should be relaxed. The examiner can confirm this by slightly moving each foot and leg before tapping with a reflex-hammer on the Achilles tendon 2 to 3 cm above the insertion at the calcaneous. He should repeat this a number of times, varying the intensity of the tap. If a positive response is present each time, the examiner should tap further away from the insertion at the calcaneous to get an estimation of the stimulus threshold. If the response is negative, the child may be asked to kneel on the chair or table with his feet dangling. The response should only be recorded as negative if no reflex response can be elicited after several trials in each position.

Response

Brief plantar flexion of the foot at the ankle may be observed. In nervous or upset children, this is sometimes accompanied by slight flexion of the knee and/or toes.

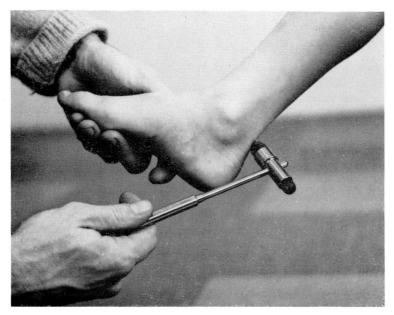

Fig. 7. Elicitation of the Achilles tendon reflex.

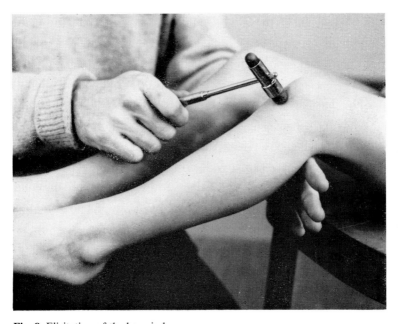

Fig. 8. Elicitation of the knee jerk.

      0 = absent
      1 = weak
      2 = moderate
      3 = brisk, sometimes followed by a few clonic beats.
      4 = sustained clonus > 7-8 beats.

Knee Jerk (Fig. 8)

Procedure

The examiner crouches in front of the child, and the child is asked to put his feet on the examiner's knees. The examiner supports the child's knees with his forearm and can confirm that the knee-muscles are relaxed by moving his arm up and down. A short tap is given on the patellar tendon ± 1 cm below the patella. It is important to check the spot as a tap slightly to the side of the tendon will often result in a non-optimal response. The examiner should attempt to elicit the response a number of times, varying the intensity of the tap, so that the responses may be compared. The stimulus threshold can be estimated by tapping at a greater distance from the patella (on or below the insertion of the quadriceps tendon at the tibia) and above the patella on the muscle itself.

Response

Quick extension of the knee caused by contraction of the quadriceps muscle may be observed. Younger children may also show a slight adductor contraction, generally in the opposite leg, but occasionally in both the opposite and the stimulated leg. The presence of any adductor contraction should be recorded separately for each side. Three-year-old children may sometimes show some hip flexion.

Recording

      0 = absent
      1 = weak
      2 = moderate
      3 = exaggerated response, sometimes followed by a few clonic beats and/or adduction of the opposite and/or stimulated leg.
      4 = sustained clonus; evident adduction of both legs.

If the knee jerk turns out to be pendular, this is recorded separately.

Biceps Reflex (Fig. 9)

Procedure

The child sits with his flexed forearm in a neutral position between pronation and supination resting along the examiner's forearm. The examiner places a finger of his supporting hand on the tendon of the child's biceps muscle, and gives the finger a short tap with the reflex-hammer. The test should be repeated with taps of varying intensity. The stimulus threshold for the reflex can be estimated by tapping higher up the upper arm along the biceps tendon and on the muscle bulk and by tapping

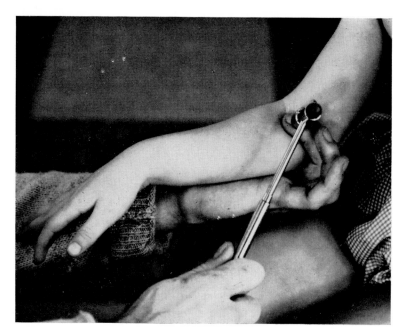

Fig. 9. Elicitation of the biceps reflex.

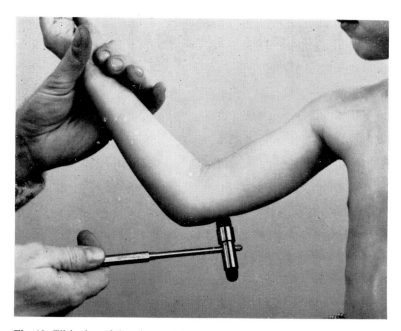

Fig. 10. Elicitation of the triceps reflex.

on the lower arm, along the volar side. For a comparison of the results on both sides, the position of the arms during the elicitation of the reflex must be symmetrical.

Response
    A quick flexion of the elbow, caused by the contraction of the biceps muscle, may be seen and/or felt. Often the brachialis muscle also contracts and the response (flexion of the forearm) is more evident. If the brachialis radialis muscle (situated at the radial side of the forearm and the biceps tendon) is stimulated, a slight pronation of the forearm may occur. In many children, especially if the forearm is kept supinated, a gentle flexion of the fingers may be seen; this response, which means a spreading of the stimulus to other muscles, is not necessarily present.

Recording
> 0 = absent.
> 1 = weak, only felt.
> 2 = moderate movements of elbow, often slight flexion of the fingers and/ or slight pronation of the forearm.
> 3 = exaggerated response; sometimes a few clonic beats; generally a marked flexion of the fingers whether the forearm is kept supinated or not.

Triceps Reflex (Fig. 10)
Procedure
    The examiner takes the child's wrist in one hand so that the elbow is semiflexed and confirms that the elbow and shoulder muscles are relaxed by gently moving these joints. He taps with the reflex-hammer on the tendon of the triceps muscle, 1 to 2 cm above the olecranon. The test should be repeated with taps of varying intensity. The stimulus threshold of the reflex can be estimated by tapping the tendon and muscle at a greater distance from the olecranon.

Response
    Quick slight extension of the elbow caused by contraction of the triceps muscle may be observed.

Recording
> 0 = absent.
> 1 = weak, only felt.
> 2 = moderate, visible movement of elbow.
> 3 = exaggerated response; clonic beats are only very rarely found; some- times a slight extension of the fingers.

Threshold of Tendon Reflexes
    As each reflex is tested, the intensity of the stimulus in the standardized position is varied. If the reflex response is found to be of high intensity or if a weak stimulus is sufficient to elicit the response, the extent of the area from which the reflex is elicitable is further explored.

The examiner faces two main problems: how many trials should be made before the reflex can be considered absent, and which intensity of response out of several trials should be recorded? If no reflex response has been elicited after 4-5 trials in a good standardized neutral position with stimuli of varying intensity, and the child's muscles are quite relaxed, then a 0 score can be given. In all cases, at least three immediately comparable responses are required for the eventual score, the stimulus being of equal intensity.

Recording

0 = no reflex elicitable.
1 = high threshold, high intensity of stimulus necessary.
2 = medium threshold.
3 = low threshold, very low intensity of stimulus necessary, extension of area from which reflex is elicitable.

Significance

Absence or low intensity of reflexes with a high threshold may be a sign of a muscle disease, a peripheral nervous disorder or lower motor neurone disease. However, in some three and four year old children, reflexes are rather difficult to elicit and responses more variable. This often bears more relationship to their soma-type than to any basic difference in the neuro-muscular system at this age.

Exaggerated responses may be due to a lesion of the upper motor neurone. Asymmetries require further investigation as, in combination with other signs, they may originate in a hemisyndrome. Obvious asymmetries of tendon reflex responses may sometimes be present as an isolated finding. This may or may not be of clinical significance. It is possible that one asymmetrical reflex may be the first or even the only manifestation of a peripheral nervous disorder or a local muscle disease. It may also be the residual effect of a past disorder (traumata, infectious diseases with high fever, disorders of endocrine gland function).

A high intensity of a reflex is quite often correlated with a low threshold, though this is not inevitable. Children with minor nervous dysfunctions may have a low threshold for a reflex of normal intensity. The reverse may also be found.

Consistent asymmetries in thresholds only and asymmetries without an obvious lateralised pattern may be signs of minor neurological dysfunction. Where lateral dominance is well established, a slight asymmetry of the threshold for tendon reflexes may be found but need not be of clinical significance. The low threshold more often occurs on the dominant side.

Plantar Response (Fig. 11)

Procedure

The examiner holds the child's foot steady in a neutral position and scratches along the lateral side of the sole from the toes towards the heel with the point of a sharp object or a thumbnail. The stimulus should be a firm scratch, but not strong enough to elicit a withdrawal of the leg.

This technique is rather different from the classical test of the plantar response, whereby the examiner scratches along the lateral side of the sole towards the toes. This method has the drawback of terminating with the specific stimulus for the grasp reflex. Thus, a plantar flexion of the toes in this instance may indicate either a positive grasp reflex or a plantar response. Clearly, it is important to differentiate between the two, especially as a positive grasp reflex in younger children may be a manifestation of a delay in maturation of the central nervous system.

Response
Three different qualities of response in the big toe may be observed.
(*a*) A negative response; no movement of the toe as a result of the stimulus.
(*b*) A *jerky* dorsi- or plantar flexion of the big toe.
(*c*) A tonic dorsi- or plantar flexion.
In the other toes, spreading or fanning may be present.

Recording
(*a*) *Big toe*
    Dorsiflexion: 0 = no reaction
                      1 = jerky dorsiflexion
                      2 = tonic, sustained dorsiflexion
    Plantar flexion: 0 = no reaction
                      1 = jerky plantar flexion
                      2 = tonic, sustained plantar flexion
(*b*) *Other toes*   0 = no fanning
                      1 = fanning present

Significance
The optimal response is plantar flexion, although in clinical practice a 'no reaction' score may also be considered normal.

Inconsistent dorsiflexion is frequently seen in children up to the age of four or five. Sustained dorsiflexion, if it does not originate in a foot deformity (pes cavus), reflects a nervous dysfunction, especially if other signs of nervous dysfunction are also present. In the case of pes cavus, the misleading dorsiflexion of the big toe may often be apparently overcome by pushing up the head of the first metatarsal bone. However, this correcting manoeuvre may elicit a grasp response, so that clear differentiation of the ultimate movement of the big toe remains problematic.

Fanning or spreading of the small toes is frequently present in children aged five or less. In older children, however, it may be a sign of nervous dysfunction, unless it is part of a general withdrawal movement of the leg.

Asymmetries may be of great significance and require further investigation. Slight differences between the responses of the left and right foot, such as plantar flexion on one side and a negative response on the other, may be regarded as meaningful asymmetries if other slight signs of lateralization are also present. An isolated asymmetry, *i.e.* an asymmetry of the plantar responses without other non-optimal findings, is usually of no clinical significance.

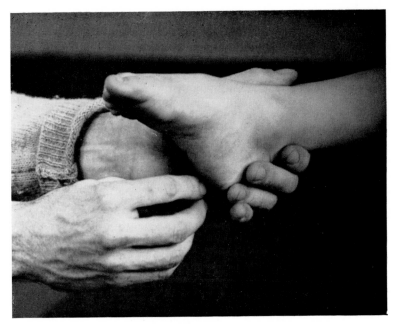

Fig. 11. Elicitation of the plantar response by scratching along the lateral side of the sole from the toes towards the heel.

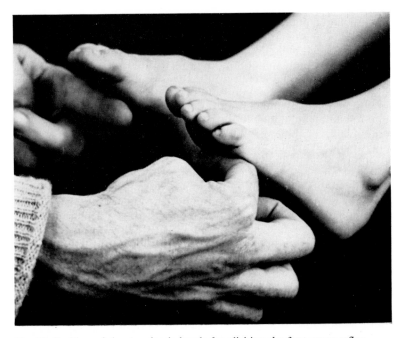

Fig. 12. Position of the examiner's hands for eliciting the foot grasp reflex.

28

Foot Grasp Reflex (Fig. 12)
Procedure
    The examiner places his index finger against the heads of the metatarsal bones, approaching them from the lateral side of the foot, and presses firmly.

Response
    Plantar flexion of all toes may be observed.

Recording
        0 = absent
        1 = weak and unsustained
        2 = sustained response for approx. 10 seconds.

Significance
    A score of 2 is always abnormal and may be a sign of delay in the maturation of the nervous system, which may occur as a retardation only, or be one of the manifestations of central nervous system damage. In cases of severe deterioration in the functioning of the central nervous system, the grasp reflex may reappear; however, this eventuality surpasses the bounds of minor nervous dysfunction.
    A score of 1 is fairly common in children under the age of four, and may be of no significance.

Palmo-mental Reflex
Procedure
    The examiner scratches along the radial side of the child's palm with a nail or a pin and observes the mental muscles of the chin.

Response
    A slight quick contraction of the homolateral musculus mentalis of the chin may be observed. In strong responses, the heterolateral muscle may also show a contraction.

Recording
        0 = absent
        1 = barely discernable, quick contraction.
        2 = obvious contraction on the homolateral side.
        3 = obvious contraction on both sides, sometimes spreading around the
              mouth.

Significance
    The optimal score is, of course, 0, but in many children this response scores 1, though it is generally not immediately reproducible. A score of 2 may be reproducible several times and is quite often found in children aged four and less. A response scoring 3 is rarely seen under normal conditions. Persistence is a sign of developmental retardation of the nervous system.

CHAPTER 4

Assessment of the Child Standing

Behavioural State

The optimal state of the child for the following series of tests is 0, though the tests may be continued if it is 1.

Position

For this series of tests, the child is asked to stand up. He should stand relaxed with his arms hanging loosely by his side.

Age

These tests are suitable for all children aged 3 to 10.

Posture

Procedure

The examiner inspects the posture of the head, body and limbs.

Recording—Head and Trunk

Any persistent deviations from a symmetrical upright posture are described by noting the appropriate score in the relevant place on the proforma (see page 93). Special attention should be paid to deviant posture of the shoulders or pelvis, *i.e.* kyphosis or exaggerated lumbar lordosis. These conditions are visible in the fully dressed child, but should be checked when the child is undressed. A slight scoliosis may go unobserved while the child is dressed and the posture of the back must therefore be re-checked at a later stage in the examination (see abdominal skin reflex, Galant response).

Significance

A marked variation in body posture may often be observed (Figs. 13-17). A child may have round shoulders but this need not have neurological significance.

Captions to Figs. 13-18 on facing page:

Fig. 13. A three-year-old child stands broad-based in a rather 'plump' fashion.

Fig. 14. The healthy five-year-old child can hold his body straight; his base is narrower and the 'plump' posture of the three-year-old has disappeared.

Fig. 15. The same child seen from the side.

Fig. 16. Standing posture of a slender seven-year-old girl with no neurological abnormalities. Note the kyphosis and lumbar lordosis.

Fig. 17. The same girl after being asked to straighten her back. Note the exaggerated lumbar lordosis.

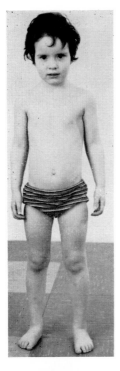 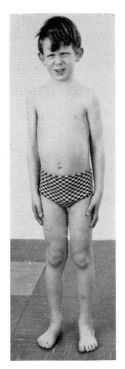 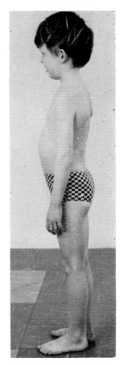

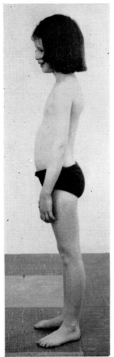 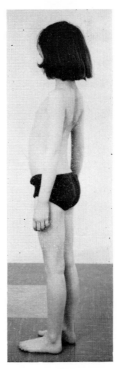

Figs. 13 - 17. Standing posture at different ages.

31

A kyphosis and exaggerated lumbar lordosis may result from static defects or from generalized muscular hypotonia, except in the case of slender young girls who often show exaggerated lumbar lordosis without any neurological significance.

An asymmetry may be part of a hemisyndrome in which the trunk and/or extremities are involved. In the case of scoliosis, a skeletal anomaly should be suspected, though it may originate from a unilateral muscular weakness (poliomyelitis) or hypertonia (irritative processes, myositis, intercostal neuritis, neoplasm (renal)). A paediatric examination is often necessary to exclude the possibility of internal diseases. There is a possibility that, in very rare cases, scoliosis may be one of the first manifest signs of Friedreich's ataxia.

Recording—Upper Limbs

The posture of the freely hanging arms is described by noting the appropriate score in the relevant box on the proforma. Exorotation, endorotation, flexion, extension, adduction and abduction are scored on a scale ranging from 0 to 2, 0 indicating that the description is not valid, 2 that the description is manifestly valid. Each side of the body is scored separately on the corresponding side of the proforma, so that both symmetrical and asymmetrical deviations can be described. In normal posture, the arms are loosely extended and slightly adducted.

Significance

An asymmetry may be part of a hemisyndrome involving the upper extremities only or the whole body. It may originate from hypertonia or hypotonia; the latter may be due to a peripheral lesion (*e.g.* a plexus paresis), muscle diseases or a dysfunction of the upper motor neurone. Static abnormalities must be excluded.

Recording—Lower Limbs

The posture of the legs and feet is recorded on the proforma, each side being scored separately so that both symmetrical and asymmetrical deviations can be described. Special attention should be paid to the width between the feet required for standing with good balance. The symmetry of the arches of the feet is also inspected and recorded.

Significance

Some degree of genu valgus is usual in children below the age of six, and is accompanied by walking and standing on the instep of the foot. The child may thus give the impression of being flat-footed, but if the ankle joint is corrected, the arch often turns out to be sufficient (Figs. 18 and 19). Normal children may vary greatly in this respect, due to the laxity of the ligaments of the joints. Extreme genu and/or pes valgus may sometimes have a neurological cause (hypotonia).

Asymmetries are generally more significant and may be due to static or neurological causes. Accidents resulting in a fractured lower leg or a sprained ankle may lead to slight asymmetry in posture long after recovery. An asymmetry may also be part of a hemisyndrome. Peripheral nervous disorder may be the cause of a unilateral collapsed arch and deviant foot posture. An abnormally large distance between the

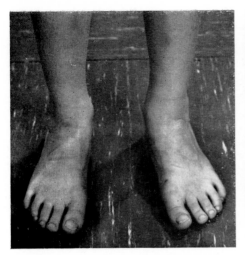 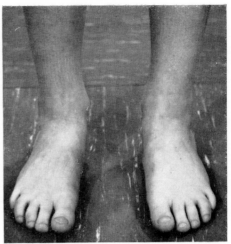

Fig. 18. The feet of a five-year-old child standing on his instep. The arch of the foot appears to be absent. After correction of the posture of the ankle joint, the arch seemed to be adequate.

Fig. 19. Flat feet in an eight-year-old child with no neurological abnormalities. After correction of the posture of the ankle joint, the arch of the foot remained inadequate.

ankles may be a sign of cerebellar or sensory dysfunction.

An extensive discussion of pes cavus and other foot deformities which accompany severe neurological diseases falls outside the scope of this book. It is well known that pes cavus may be part of, or even the only manifestation of a status dysraphicus, and on rare occasions it may be the first sign of a Friedreich's ataxia.

Spontaneous Motility

Procedure

Spontaneous motor activity is observed in the same way as in the sitting position (see page 11). A distinction is made between gross and small motor movements, and the quantity and quality of each type of movement are recorded separately. Special attention should be paid to the occurrence of involuntary movements (see page 36).

As the child is at this point standing and waiting for things to happen, it may be difficult to assess the quality of movement. However, during the observation of posture, the child may be asked to stand up straight, relax, turn round, *etc.*, and the movements needed for these actions can be observed for their quality.

Observation of motor activity in the standing position is principally concerned with gross movements, while observation in the sitting position is also concerned with minor movements such as playing with and manipulating toys.

Recording

(*a*) *Quantity*

Gross movements: 0 = no movements. The child stands perfectly still for at least 2 minutes.

33

1 = a few movements only. The child stays in the same place, but turns round slightly, shifts his feet, moves his arms, etc.

2 = a moderate amount of movements. The child still stays in more or less the same place, but turns round, bends down, then straightens up again, turns his head round several times, moves his arms, etc.

3 = an excessive amount of movements. The child cannot stay in the same place and continuously moves his body, head and/or limbs.

Small movements: 0 = no movements. The child stands perfectly still without moving hands, feet or facial musculature, etc.

1 = a few movements only, mainly of the hands and face.

2 = a moderate amount of movements. The child opens and closes his hands, pulls faces from time to time wiggles his toes, fidgets with his clothes, etc.

3 = an excessive amount of movements. The child moves and fidgets all the time, makes faces and plucks at his clothes continuously, etc.

(b) *Quality*

Speed: 0 = the child stands perfectly still.

1 = the movements are performed slowly.

2 = the movements are performed at a moderate tempo.

3 = all movements are performed very rapidly.

Smoothness: 0 = the child stands perfectly still.

1 = all movements are very smooth and supple.

2 = movements are mostly smooth and supple, often depending on their speed.

3 = movements are performed clumsily and may be abrupt and jerky, often giving the impression of being broken down into constituent parts.

4 = all movements are performed very awkwardly or are very abrupt and jerky.

Adequacy: 0 = the child stands perfectly still.

1 = movements are easily goal-directed.

2 = some movements are goal-directed, others are inadequate and do not serve a clear purpose.

3 = the child moves around aimlessly; his movements are mainly inadequate.

(c) *Involuntary movements*

Type and localisation are described if present (see page 36).

Significance

A score of 3 for the quantity of movements describes overactivity, but such a description does not indicate a diagnosis. Some children may be hyperactive during

34

certain parts of the examination and quiet and attentive for the rest of the time. Others may be active all the time, and in these cases an observation of the quality of movements may well indicate a rather abrupt and jerky motion. We feel that children with very jerky movements are often those with a hyperkinetic syndrome associated with true cerebral dysfunction, while children whose hyperactivity is an environmental phenomenon show movements of a different quality. We have not yet been able to differentiate quality of movement effectively in enough children to be certain of this, but we do believe that it is worthwhile attempting to describe quality as well as quantity of movement.

Other signs of neurological dysfunction, such as dyskinesia, difficulties of co-ordination or a high amount of associated movements, may often be observed at the same time. Clumsy children may show a low amount of spontaneous movements, and often their speed of movement is low. This is particularly true of children aged less than six.

Posture with Arms Extended (Figs. 20 and 21)

Procedure

The child is asked to stand with his feet together and his head centred, and then to stretch out his arms, palms downwards, for twenty seconds. The test is repeated with the palms turned upwards (in supination). Children aged six and over should be asked to close their eyes during the test.

Fig. 20 (left). Standing with arms extended and pronated.
Fig. 21 (right). Standing with arms extended and supinated.

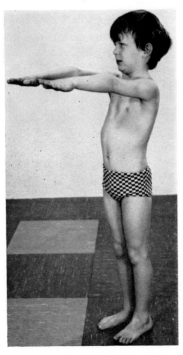 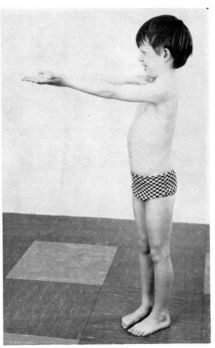

35

Recording

Lateral and vertical deviations from the median line are recorded. The degree of pronation which occurs after the hands have been held in supination for some time is also recorded.

The posture of the wrist joints should be noted, as often the hand and forearm are not perfectly aligned. There may be a kind of double angle, the wrist being somewhat flexed and the fingers hyperextended in the metacarpal phalangeal joints; this is known as fork-posture or 'spooning'.

Deviation from horizontal line: 0 = no deviation
1 = arms drop
2 = arms rise

Deviation from the median line: 0 = no deviation
1 = 30° to 60° sidewards
2 = 60° to 90° sidewards

Spooning: 0 = no spooning
1 = minimal spooning
2 = obvious spooning

Pronation: 0 = no pronation
1 = pronation over 30° to 60°
2 = pronation over 60° to 90°

Each side is scored separately.

Significance

A slight horizontal deviation is common in children below the age of six, usually in an upward direction if the arms are kept pronated, and downwards if the arms are kept in supination (Figs. 22 and 23). Also, a slight deviation from the median line may be observed in this age-group; in three-year-old children often up to score 1 (Fig. 23). In slender children, in particular, some degree of spooning is often present, generally in both arms. In such cases, there is often a slightly increased range of movements in wrist and finger joints (Fig. 24). A score of 1 for pronation of out-stretched supinated arms is common in children aged less than five. However, children aged three and four may not do this test reliably.

Asymmetries may be the result of a hemisyndrome or other unilateral functional disturbances, *e.g.* sensorimotor innervation disturbances, unilateral co-ordination difficulties or local disorders (post-traumatic residual state, muscle or joint diseases, *etc.*). However, a strongly expressed hand dominance may also account for slight asymmetries, usually in the non-dominant hand.

TESTS FOR INVOLUNTARY MOVEMENTS

Behavioural State

These tests can only be carried out if the child's state is 0.

Age

These tests are difficult to carry out on children aged less than four.

36

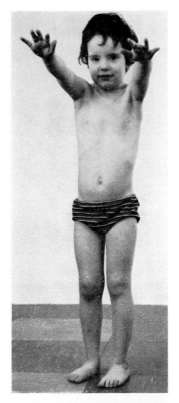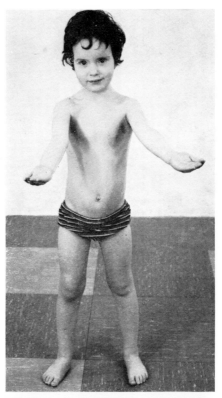

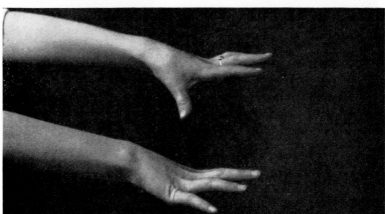

Fig. 22 (above left). A normal three-year-old girl standing with arms extended and pronated. Note the upward deviation of the arms. A slight deviation to the side is also present.

Fig. 23 (above right). The same child standing with arms extended and supinated. There is now a downward deviation and again a slight deviation to the side.

Fig. 24 (below). 'Spooning' of the wrists and hands in a five-year-old girl. When the arms are extended, the wrist joints are slightly flexed and the fingers hyperextended in the metacarpophalangeal joints.

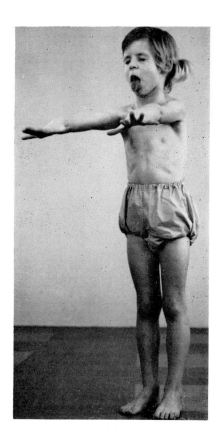

Fig. 25. Posture for tests of involuntary movements in older children.

Procedure

The child is asked to stand with his feet together and his head centred, and then to stretch out his arms with his fingers spread as wide apart as possible, keeping them still for twenty seconds (Fig. 25). Children aged six and over are asked to close their eyes tightly and to stick out their tongue; younger children may be allowed to keep their eyes open, as they are easily frightened when their eyes are closed. The test must be standardized for age, so that comparisons between the same age groups can be made.

It is important that the child should put the maximum effort into spreading his fingers as wide as possible, as slight involuntary movements are often only seen in this position.

General Remarks

The words athetoid and athetotic are extremely misleading; sometimes they are used synonymously and sometimes they are attributed distinct meanings. We have attempted here to give a precise operational definition of what we understand by certain terms in every instance. Where more than one term is used synonymously in the literature we have listed the alternatives but feel that many authors are imprecise in their use of such terms. The fact that one type of movement shows some resemblance

38

to another type of movement does not mean that both types of movement are etio-logically or pathogenetically identical *e.g.* choreatic and choreiform movements.

Choreiform Movements (syn.: choreatiform movements)
These are small jerky movements which occur quite irregularly and arhythmically in different muscles. They may occur in all muscles of the body and can be recorded electromyographically in relaxed muscles, where they are not visible on gross inspection.

The examiner should look for choreiform movements in fingers, and wrist joints (distal choreiform movements), and in the arms and shoulders (proximal choreiform movements (Prechtl and Stemmer 1962).

Recording
       0 = no choreiform movements visible during the 20 seconds.
       1 = 2-5 isolated twitches
       2 = 6-10 twitches, usually in bursts
       3 = continuous twitching
Distal and proximal choreiform movements are recorded separately.

Athetotiform Movements (syn.: athetoid-like movements)
These are small slow movements, rather writhing in appearance, which occur quite irregularly and arhythmically in different muscles. They presumably may occur in all muscles of the body, but are best seen in the muscles of the fingers and tongue.

In this test, the examiner should look for athetotiform movements in the fingers only.

Recording
       0 = no athetotiform movements visible during the 20 seconds.
       1 = 2-5 slow writhing movements
       2 = 6-10 slow writhing movements
       3 = continuous writhing movements

Choreo-athetotic Movements
These are usually associated with severe neurological diseases, but they are described here because of the difficulty of distinguishing them, when they are of light intensity, from less marked movements such as choreiform and athetotiform movements.

Choreatic Movements (syn.: movements of chorea)
These consist of rather gross jerky movements occurring irregularly and arhythmically in different muscles. The patient may sometimes have difficulty in keeping his balance because of their amplitude and intensity. The bursts are longer and more gross in comparison with choreiform movements. Electromyographically, choreiform movements appear as short twitches, while choreatic movements appear as bursts of activity.

Athetoid Movements (syn.: athetotic movements)

These are slow writhing movements which occur continuously, irregularly and arhythmically in different muscles. They are usually of a greater amplitude than athetotiform movements.

Athetosis and chorea are often present at the same time, and in athetotic cerebral palsy resulting from kernicterus, athetosis is rarely present without chorea.

Recording

Choreatic movements: 0 = no choreatic movements

1 = slight choreatic movements which may interfere with ordinary motor activity or posture.

2 = marked choreatic movements which seriously interfere with ordinary activities and occasionally throw the child off balance.

3 = severe choreatic movements which render ordinary activities and normal posture quite impossible.

Athetoid movements: 0 = no athetoid movements

1 = slight athetoid movements which may interfere with ordinary activities, but not conspicuously.

2 = marked athetoid movements, often in bursts, which seriously interfere with normal motor behaviour.

3 = severe athetoid movements which render ordinary activities and normal posture quite impossible.

A score of 3 for choreiform movements may resemble a score of 1 for choreatic movements. However, this does not mean that choreiform movements can be considered simply as a minor degree of choreo-athetosis.

Tremor

This consists of involuntary rhythmical alternating movements.

A clear distinction must be drawn between resting tremor and tremor which occurs during movement. In this test, the examiner should look for resting tremor only, in the fingers and forearms.

Recording

0 = no tremor present.

1 = barely discernable tremor.

2 = marked tremor of the fingers.

3 = marked tremor of the fingers and arms.

Significance

The significance of choreiform movements is still open to discussion (Rutter *et al.* 1966). However, this type of dyskinesia (Prechtl and Stemmer 1962) seems to be associated with groups of children showing different behaviour (Wolff and Hurwitz 1966) and may be seen as a sign of non-optimal nervous function. Children who do not show choreiform movements at an early age may develop them when

40

they reach the age of four or five; thus, all children in the age group under discussion should be carefully observed for such movements. Once they have emerged, they usually remain until after puberty.

There is a clear difference between the sexes, the incidence of choreiform movements being two to three times higher in boys than in girls. This is not so marked in the case of athetotiform movements, the significance of which is also less certain. This book is confined to the methodological question of how to elicit and record signs which are clearly present in order to analyse the meaning of these findings in relation to behavioural and learning difficulties. As long as the pathological significance of these phenomena is not refuted, such signs should be taken into account.

Tremor is a phenomenon which is often seen in children of school age and often appears to be 'situation-bound'. However, some types of tremor may be either of primary neurological origin (paresis, hereditary tremor) or secondary neurological origin (thyreotoxicosis, intoxications). A Parkinson-type of tremor is rarely found in children and its presence would clearly transgress the bounds of 'minor dysfunction'.

TESTS FOR COORDINATION AND ASSOCIATED MOVEMENTS

Mouth-opening Finger-spreading Phenomenon (Figs. 26 and 27)

Age

This test is suitable for all children aged 3 to 10.

Procedure

The examiner supports the child's extended arms so that the hands and wrists are relaxed. The child is asked to open his mouth as wide as he can and to close his eyes and stick out his tongue, if a greater effect is desired.

Fig. 26. Initial position of the mouth-opening finger-spreading phenomenon.

Fig. 27. Response on opening the mouth and closing the eyes.

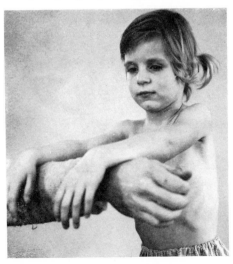
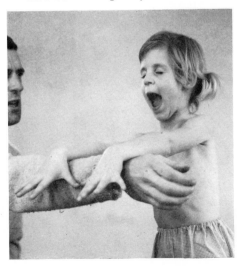

Response

Spreading and extension of the fingers may be observed.

Recording

     0 = no movements of the relaxed fingers.
     1 = barely discernible spreading.
     2 = marked spreading with some extension.
     3 = maximal spreading and often extension of all the fingers.

Significance

This phenomenon is usually present in three- to four-year-old children and decreases in intensity with age. At the age of seven or eight, the majority of children show no sign of the phenomenon except for occasional slight indications if the child is asked to close his eyes tight and stick out his tongue as far as possible. The persistance of a response in children older than eight years may be interpreted as a sign of retardation of nervous functioning.

Diadochokinesis and Associated Movements (Figs. 28 and 29)

Procedure

The child is required to stand with one arm relaxed at his side and the other flexed at an angle of over 90° at the elbow, the hand pointing forwards. The child's

Fig. 28. Diadochokinesis of the right lower arm. On supination of the right hand, associated supination occurs in the left hand.

Fig. 29. On pronation of the right hand, associated pronation occurs in the left hand. Movement of the right elbow during the diadochokinesis is clearly visible (compare with Fig. 28).

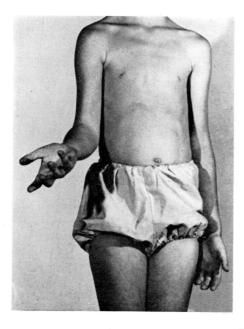

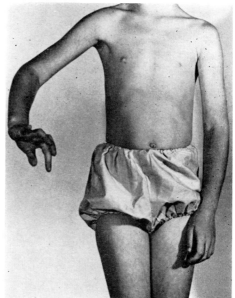

head must be centred and his arm and shoulder relaxed. Diadochokinesis consists of quickly pronating and supinating the hand and forearm. The examiner must demonstrate the movement at a speed of four complete pro- and supinations per second. He then asks the child to imitate this movement at the same speed. Abduction and adduction of the arm often occurs in children, resulting in movements of the elbow. The distance the elbow moves can be used as a measure for the diadochokinesis. If the movements of diadochokinesis are smooth but accompanied by elbow movements, the child may be re-instructed to concentrate on wrist movements but not specifically to keep the elbow still.

Associated movements should be looked for in the opposite arm. These consist mainly of mirror movements, sometimes accompanied by flexion of the elbow.

The test lasts approximately 15 seconds.

Recording

Diadochokinesis: 0 = no pro- and supination of the forearm, but other movements present.

1 = awkward pro- and supination, the elbow moving over a distance of more than 15 cm.

2 = awkward pro- and supination, the elbow moving over a distance of 5-15 cm.

3 = smooth and correctly performed pro- and supination, the elbow moving over a distance of less than 5 cm.

Associated movements: 0 = no visible mirror movements or flexion of the elbow.

1 = barely discernable mirror movements or slight flexion of the elbow without mirror movements.

2 = marked mirror movements without flexion of the elbow.

3 = marked mirror movements with flexion of the elbow.

The score for each arm is recorded separately.

Significance

A score of 1 or 2 for diadochokinesis and 2 or 3 for associated movements is quite common in very young children. At the age of six and seven years, the usual score is 2 in both instances, while at the age of eight and over pro- and supination of the forearm is generally smooth and accompanied by a decreased amount of associated movements. Sometimes at this age a flexion of the elbow may be seen in the opposite arm without any mirror movements in the hand.

If this test is carried out when the child is sitting down, mirror movements in the legs and feet may also be observed. However, since it is difficult for a single observer to score all these at the same time, and since hand and arm movements are best observed when the child is standing, we decided to concentrate on associated movements in the upper limbs. Quite often an asymmetry between the diadochokinesis and the associated movements on the two sides of the body may be observed. Such a discrepancy between the functioning of the right and left arm often increases with age, the pro- and supination improving at a faster rate on the dominant side. Similarly, the amount of associated movements may decrease at different rates on the two sides as the child grows older. In a child with a clearly established dominance, associated movements may occur on the dominant side when the non-dominant arm is moving. However, when dominance is not so firmly established, associated movements may sometimes be seen to a greater degree in the non-dominant arm.

The appearance of associated movements is also governed by several other factors. The order in which the hands are tested may influence the results, and the effects of learning and practice of skilled and complex movements are uncertain. It is advisable to carry out a preliminary trial for 15 seconds to acquaint the child with the test, and to record his scores on his second attempt.

An asymmetrical performance may be interpreted as an indication of lateralisation or a hemisyndrome only if other neurological test items corroborate such an interpretation.

A low score for diadochokinesis and a high score for associated movements in children aged ten and over may be seen as a sign of retarded maturation of these nervous functions.

When dysdiadochokinesis is the result of cerebellar dysfunction, the movements of pro- and supination are more awkward, incomplete and slow, and they seem to be broken down into single movements which tend to overshoot. A rate of four complete pro- and supinations per second is usually not possible.

Finger-nose Test (Figs. 30 and 31)
Age
This test is routinely appropriate for children aged over 4 to 5 only.

Fig. 30 (left). The child moves his index finger to his nose, keeping his eyes closed.
Fig. 31 (right). He keeps his fingertip on the tip of his nose for a few moments before reopening his eyes.

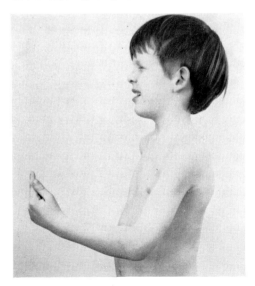
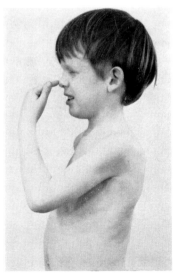

Procedure

The child is asked to put the tip of his index finger (*i.e.* the distal finger-pulpa) on the tip of his nose. The movement must be carried out slowly. The test is repeated three times with each hand; children aged five may be asked to repeat the test with their eyes closed, but we feel that this might upset younger children.

The examiner must demonstrate the test as he gives the instructions. Some children may still persist in putting their finger on the side of their nose, or touching the bridge of the nose. In these cases, the examiner may take hold of the child's finger and place it correctly on the child's nose, so that the child understands what he is required to do. Sometimes, though rarely, the test must be turned into a game as with a doll ('touch the doll's nose, touch your own nose'). This should not be necessary if the examiner has established a good relationship with the child.

Recording

The test is scored twice, once for the quality, *i.e.* the smoothness of the movements and signs of intention tremor, and once for adequacy, *i.e.* success in placing the fingertip on the tip of the nose.

Smoothness: 0 = no tremor present during the movement.
1 = slight tremor, occurring only at the end of the movement.
2 = marked tremor, increasing towards the end of the movement.

N.B. Tremor is defined here as an oscillating movement of the finger, sometimes of the whole hand, occurring during the movement of the arm. It may be quite irregular and arythmical.

Adequacy: 0 = the child puts his fingertip correctly on the tip of his nose each time.
1 = the child misses the tip of his nose once or twice.
2 = the child misses the tip of his nose each time.

Consistent deviations or misplacings to one side are also described.

Significance

When this test is performed with eyes closed, it is a test of cerebellar function, but the sensory system (proprioceptors) is also involved. If the child keeps his eyes open, visual guidance of the movements provides additional information which is often essential for children aged less than five (Figs. 32 and 33).

Slight difficulties in performing the test, indicated by scores of 2, presumably reflect proprioceptive rather than cerebellar functions. However, there is a possibility that they may be the first manifestation of a progressive cerebellar disease.

Fingertip-touching Test (Figs. 34 and 35)

Age

This test is suitable for all children aged 3 to 10, but can only be performed with eyes closed by children aged 7 and over.

45

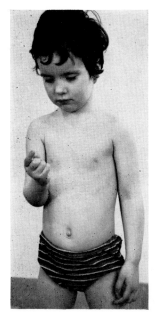
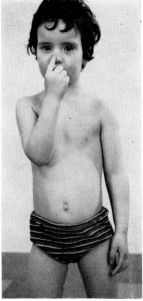

Fig. 32. The finger-nose test in a cooperative three-year-old girl. Visual guidance of the finger movement is necessary.

Fig. 33. Visual guidance is no longer necessary when the goal has been achieved. Note the difference in arm posture compared with Fig. 31; the younger child needs to hold her arm against her body for stabilisation.

Procedure

The examiner stands in front of the child and points an index finger at him, keeping his elbow flexed. The child is asked to put the tip of his index finger on the tip of the examiner's finger, the distance between them being such that the child has to flex his elbow to accomplish this. The test is carried out three times with each hand, first with eyes open and then with eyes closed. The examiner must take care not to change the position of his finger.

Fig. 34. Training procedure for the fingertip-touching test in a seven-year-old girl; the eyes are open.

Fig. 35. Response with eyes closed in the same girl.

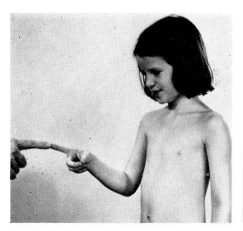
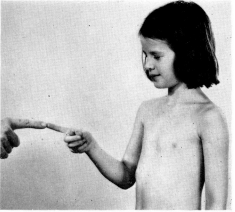

46

Recording

The test is scored for quality, *i.e.* intention tremor during movement and when the finger is placed, and adequacy, *i.e.* success in placing the fingertip on the examiner's finger. Separate recordings are made when the eyes are open and when the eyes are closed.

Tremor during movement: 0 = no tremor present
            1 = slight tremor
            2 = marked tremor

Tremor of the placed finger: 0 = no tremor present
            1 = slight tremor
            2 = marked tremor

Placing the finger: 0 = the child places his finger correctly on the examiner's fingertip each time.
            1 = the child misses once or twice.
            2 = the child misses each time.

Consistent deviations and misplacings to one side are also described.

Significance

The optimal response is a smooth and adequate placing of the finger on the examiner's fingertip. When carried out with eyes open, both cerebellar and proprioceptive sensory systems are involved. When carried out with eyes closed, it is mainly a test of proprioception. A score of 1 in placing of the finger with closed eyes is usual in children up to 7-8 years of age. Older children should, on the whole, perform better. Any tremor during movement, particularly if it increases towards completion of the movement, should arouse the suspicion of ataxia (intention tremor). This kind of tremor is usually rather coarse and irregular. A regular, rather fine tremor, commonly called 'psychogenic tremor', may frequently be observed while the child's finger rests on the examiner's finger, and seems to have no clinical significance.

Consistent deviations to one side may reflect a unilateral cerebellar or vestibular dysfunction.

Finger Opposition Test

Age

This test is applicable to most children of 6 years and older. Some agile 5 year olds are also able to perform it smoothly.

Procedure

The examiner demonstrates to the child how to place the fingers of one hand consecutively on the thumb of the same hand, starting with the index finger in the sequence: 2, 3, 4, 5, 4, 3, 2, 3, 4, 5, etc. The child is asked to imitate these movements, completing five sequences to and fro. Each hand is tested in turn. The test should be carried out at a rate of approximately 3 to 4 seconds for one complete sequence.

47

Recording

This test is scored on three aspects: the smoothness of movement, governed by hesitations in correcting mistakes and associated movements in the other fingers of the same hand; smoothness of transition from one finger to the next, especially at the turning-points involving the index and the little fingers; and mirror movements, *i.e.* associated movements in the opposite hand.

Smoothness of movement:	0 = smooth placing of fingers on the thumb.
	1 = slightly clumsy movement. The child hesitates, sometimes misplaces a finger, gets the sequence wrong or wiggles a finger before placing it.
	2 = many hesitations and misplacings with associated movements of other fingers which hamper adequate placing.
Finger-to-finger transition:	0 = easy and immediate transition.
	1 = the child puts the same finger on the thumb several times at the turn.
	2 = the child repeatedly puts a finger on the thumb before going on to the next finger.
	3 = the child repeatedly puts a finger on the thumb, even when he wants to go on to the next finger.
Mirror movements:	0 = no associated movements in the opposite hand.
	1 = barely discernable associated movements.
	2 = marked associated movements.

Significance

Most children aged six and over can perform this test, a score of 0 or 1 for finger-to-finger transition and smoothness of movement being possible in normal children at the age of eight. A score of 1 for mirror movements may be present up to 10 years. Girls often manage this test better than boys. As with diadochokinesis, the finger-opposition test may be impaired when other manual coordination tests such as the fingertip-nose and fingertip-touching tests are performed quite adequately. Naturally, hand dominance is an important factor in the quality of the performance. Learning is also important, and it is advisable to let the child practise five sequences before his performance is scored. The examiner must make quite sure that the child understands what he is expected to do before the test begins, since young children often find difficulty with this test.

During the test, mirror movements in the other hand may sometimes be seen, and these may reflect a retarded maturation of the nervous system. Most children aged ten and over do not show mirror movements on this test, and girls generally show fewer associated movements than boys.

48

Standing with Eyes Closed

Procedure

The child is asked to keep his eyes closed for ten to fifteen seconds. With very young children aged three to four it may be necessary to invent a game, *e.g.* 'Let's see how long you can stand still with your eyes closed. Close your eyes and I shall count how long you can do it.'

Recording

As this is a test of balance, *i.e.* the ability to maintain equilibrium without visual control, the amount of movement of body, arms, legs and feet needed for this purpose is recorded.

0 = no balance with eyes closed. The child has to step to one side in order to prevent himself falling.

1 = balance is only possible with the aid of movements of the whole body, often resulting in a slight shifting of the feet.

2 = balance is possible with the aid of only a few movements of the ankles and toes.

3 = perfect balance and no movements.

A consistent tendency to fall to one side is recorded.

Significance

Slight swaying movements of the body unaccompanied by isolated arm or leg movements are often seen, especially at the end of the time limit, and do not seem to have any clinical significance.

Children aged less than six often need a few movements of ankles and toes to maintain balance, without any actual displacement of the feet, and this also appears to be without clinical significance.

Quite often, involuntary movements may interfere with optimal performance and this should be taken into account in the final interpretation of the findings.

A tendency to fall to one side may be a sign of unilateral vestibular or cerebellar dysfunction. A lack of balance without consistent laterality often reflects retardation of maturation, a muscular weakness or intensive dyskinesia.

CHAPTER 5

Assessment of the Child Walking

Behavioural State

The optimal state of the child for the following series of tests is 0, though the tests are possible if it is 1 or 2.

Position

The child is asked to stand with his head straight and his arms by his sides.

Age

These tests are suitable for all children aged 3 to 10, except where indicated.

Gait (Fig. 36)
Procedure

The child is asked to walk over a distance of approximately 20 continuous paces and back. He should be relaxed and walk quietly at a normal pace. The examiner must look out for acting.

Fig. 36. Walking.

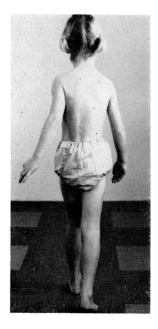

Recording

The posture of head, body and arms during walking is recorded (see scoring criteria, page 10). Special attention should also be paid to the width of gait, movements of the arms and movements of the hips and knees. If flexion of the hip, knee and/or ankle is impaired on one side, the child will compensate for this by circumducting the leg in an arc away from the hip. (In extreme cases such as spastic hemiplegia with equinovarus posture of the foot, the pelvis will be raised on the affected side and the toes may still scrape against the floor.) This is known as 'circumduction' of the leg. The examiner should also take note of the way in which the feet are placed. In normal gait, the heel touches the ground first and weight is then shifted to the toes with an arching of the foot. This is referred to as the 'heel-toe' gait.

It may happen that asymmetries or other deviations of posture present when the child is standing (resulting, for instance, from slight scoliosis, slight diffuse hypotonia or asymmetrical, mainly static, foot posture) may disappear during walking. The reverse may also be the case. These phenomena should be described.

Width of gait:	0 = constant
	1 = variable
	0 = < 10 cm.
	1 = 11-20 cm.
	2 = 21-30 cm.
	3 = > 30 cm.
Circumduction:	0 = no circumduction
	1 = barely discernable (left and/or right)
	2 = marked (left and/or right)
Movements of pelvis:	0 = short abrupt movements
	1 = swinging movements
	2 = dipping movements
Movements of the knees:	0 = alternating flexion/extension
	1 = constantly flexed
	2 = constantly extended
Heel-toe gait:	0 = no heel-toe gait, no arching of the foot
	1 = heel-toe gait, but no evident arching of the foot
	2 = heel-toe gait, marked arching of the foot.
Arm movements:	0 = normal swing
	1 = arms hanging down without any active movement
	2 = arms kept in abduction
	3 = arms kept in adduction
Placing of the feet:	Each foot is scored separately for abduction, adduction, dorsiflexion and plantar flexion on the medial and lateral side.

In difficult cases, Holt's footprint method (1965) may be useful.

Significance

Asymmetries in the posture of the head or body during walking may be due to neurological or orthopaedic causes (*e.g.* hemiplegia, flat feet or rheumatoid arthritis). In cases of generalised hypotonia, the posture may be symmetrical but abnormal. Asymmetries in arm or leg movements may be signs of a mild lateralisation or hemi-syndrome.

Children below the age of six quite often show only minimal arching of the foot, and in extreme cases the foot may even be endorotated and pronated. Often these children cannot walk long distances and are easily tired on walking trips. Generally no arching of the foot is visible while the child is standing still. A perpendicular from the internal malleolus reaching the floor outside the circumference of the footprint indicates talipes valgus (see Fig. 18, page 33). At this age, this is usually a result of lax ligaments around the ankle joints, and postural deviations generally disappear during the course of the next few years as the ligaments grow stronger. There may be a neurological cause such as hypotonia, but this is rare. Most so-called 'flat feet' at this age are really talipes valgus disorders. Treatment with arch supports, which does not act causally, is of little value; the ideal treatment is the introduction of strong shoes that support the ankle joint and counteract the tendency to walk on the instep. Asymmetries and extreme cases of symmetrical talipes valgus must be carefully examined as they may be of neurological origin (*e.g.* lateralisations, hypotonia, isolated hypertonia.)

Children below the age of five tend to show only a few arm movements while walking, the four-year-old generally keeping his arms still.

In children over the age of six, arching of the foot should be evident during walking, and should generally be visible while standing. Pes planus should be suspected if the posture of the ankle joint is adequate, but no arching of the foot is visible (see Fig. 19, page 33). Again, in most cases static or perhaps hereditary factors are important. In cases of marked pes planus, a symmetrical abduction posture of the feet is customary.

Circumduction of one leg results from inadequate integration of knee and/or ankle movements in locomotion, and may be due to nervous dysfunction, such as spastic hemiparesis, or to arthrogenic or mygenic causes. In cases of mild hypertonia on one side of the body, circumduction may be evident before the examination of the resistance against passive movements reveals any clearcut difference between the two legs. This must be differentiated from the effects of pain which, by immobilising joints, may also lead to some degree of circumduction.

In normal gait, the distance between the feet remains constant. A variable width of gait may be arthrogenic (*e.g.* luxation or subluxation of the hip joint) or neurological in origin, although once again this must be differentiated from a variable width of gait due to pain.

In very young children (two to three years) slight asymmetries of gait may be observed unaccompanied by other signs of neurological dysfunction. It is possible that in these cases a certain degree of plagiocephaly (asymmetry of the skull, generally the result of postnatal head posture) may be present (Robson 1968). Children of three to four years may also show similar asymmetries of gait without evidence of other neurological dysfunction, but these usually disappear as the child grows older. Arthrogenic or static causes may be found in some of these children, but even if no such causes can be diagnosed, the clinical significance of such an isolated finding is doubtful.

The normal width of gait in children over three years is 11 to 20 cm. A markedly narrow width of gait may result from hypertonia of the adductor muscles of the leg. A wide width of gait may be caused by nervous dysfunction (*e.g.* muscular hypotonia of the leg and/or pelvic girdle, sensory or cerebellar dysfunction) or may be arthrogenic in origin as in the case of luxation or subluxation of the hip joint.

It must be borne in mind that the posture of the feet may vary considerably in the individual during walking, and that findings may therefore be rather difficult to interpret. Marked exo- or endorotation or marked dorsi- or plantar flexion should arouse the suspicion of abnormality, as should any marked asymmetries. However, as with other signs, clearly a final interpretation can only be made when the examination has been completed.

Walking along a Straight Line
Age
This test is applicable to children aged 5 to 10 years.

Procedure
The child is asked to walk along a straight line over a distance of approximately 20 continuous paces and back again. He is not required to place one foot directly in front of the other.

Recording
The number of deviations from the line is counted.
0 = the child cannot walk three steps successively without deviating from the line.
1 = 6 deviations.
2 = 4-6 deviations.
3 = no deviations.
A consistent deviation to one side should be noted.

Significance
Between the ages of five and seven, three deviations are acceptable. Poor performance may be due to hypotonia, hypertonia, cerebellar or sensory dysfunction. Involuntary movements, such as choreiform movements or tremor, may interfere with optimal performance. Persistent difficulties may reflect a hemisyndrome.

Walking on Tiptoe (Fig. 37)
Procedure
The child is asked to walk on tiptoe over a distance of approximately 20 continuous paces and back.

Recording
0 = unable to walk on tiptoe.
1 = heel raised for only a few moments.
2 = the heel remains off the ground.
3 = the child walks well on tiptoe.
Any movements of the head, body or arms which are not present in ordinary walking must be noted as associated movements; this does not include ordinary slight swinging of the arms, for instance. Associated movements are most clearly seen in the arms and face. The arms and hands generally extend and lip and tongue movements may be present. Clenched fists may be seen, but these are only considered as associated movements if they are accompanied by extended arms.
0 = no associated movements visible.
1 = barely discernable associated movements in the arms and hands only.
2 = marked extension of the arms and hands, or extension of the arms with clenched fists.
3 = as for '2', with abduction of the upper arms and/or lip and tongue movements.

Children over three should be able to walk on tiptoe; some younger children are also able to do so, but if they cannot no abnormality is indicated. Poor performance may be due to hypotonia or flexor hypertonia, while a high score may be due to extensor hypertonia. Asymmetries may be a sign of a lateralisation syndrome and should be carefully investigated; unilateral foot deformities and other non-neurological causes must clearly first be eliminated. Bilateral foot deformities may also influence performance.

The amount of associated movements decreases with age and should have disappeared by the age of seven or eight. The persistence of associated movements may be one aspect of slow neurological development.

Walking on Heels (Fig. 38)

Procedure

The child is asked to walk on his heels over a distance of approximately 20 continuous paces and back.

Recording

      0 = unable to walk on heels.
      1 = toes raised for only a few moments.
      2 = the toes remain off the ground.
      3 = the child walks well on the dorsal half of the heels.

Any movements of the head, body or arms which are not present in ordinary walking must be noted as associated movements; these are most clearly seen in the arms and face, when present. Generally the arms flex at the elbows, the wrists hyperextend and the fingers flex at the interphalangeal joints; the fingers may also be extended. Quite often the upper arms are abducted at the shoulder joint, and lip and/or tongue movements may be observed.

      0 = no associated movements visible.
      1 = barely discernable flexion of the elbows and hyperextension of the wrists.
      2 = marked flexion of the elbows (up to 60°) and hyperextension of the wrists.
      3 = As for '2' (elbow flexion > 60°) with abduction of the shoulders and/or movements of lips and tongue.

Significance

Children over three should be able to walk on their heels; some younger children may already be able to do so. Poor performance may be due to hypotonia of the lower leg muscles or paresis. It is of particular interest that paresis of the peroneal muscles may occur without other muscles being impaired to the same degree. The child will walk on the outer side of the foot rather than on the heels, or, in mild cases, will commence on the heel but fail soon afterwards and walk on endorotated feet. Clearly, any foot deformities will interfere with performance. Asymmetries may indicate a

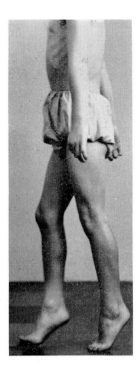
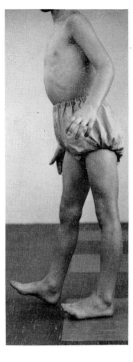

Fig. 37. Walking on tiptoe. Slight extension of the elbows is present.

Fig. 38. Walking on heels. Marked associated movements are visible (flexion of the elbow, slight hyper-extension of the wrist, extension and spreading of the fingers).

Fig. 39. Standing on the left leg.   **Fig. 40.** Hopping on the right leg.

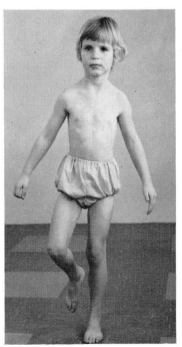
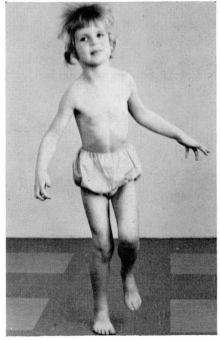

lateralisation syndrome or they may result from non-neurological causes (*e.g.* unilateral foot deformities, arthrogenic origins, etc.).

Associated movements accompanying walking on heels persist longer than in the case of walking on tiptoe, but generally disappear by the age of nine or ten. The persistence of associated movements at this age may be interpreted as a sign of slow neurological development.

Standing on One Leg (Fig. 39)

Procedure

The child is asked to stand on one leg for at least 20 seconds. Each leg is tested in turn, the child being allowed to start with whichever leg he prefers.

Recording

The performance of each leg is recorded separately and a note is made of which leg the child uses first.

$0 =$ unable to stand on one leg.
$1 =$ tries, but has to put foot down again.
$2 =$ 3-6 secs.
$3 =$ 7-12 secs.
$4 =$ 13-16 secs.
$5 =$ 17-20 secs.
$6 =$ more than 20 secs. This is regarded as a mature performance.

Significance

The ability to stand on one leg develops quite suddenly and improves rapidly. At three years of age only a few children can stand on one leg for longer than 5 to 6 seconds; at five years, most children can carry on for 10 to 12 seconds; at six, 13 to 16 seconds is normal; and by the age of seven or eight, most children are able to stand on one leg for more than 20 seconds.

The difference between the performance of the preferred and the non-preferred leg is greatest at the age of four and five and decreases with age. At the age of three or four, a score of 1 or 2 is usual. At this age also, many 'balancing' movements are needed. In children older than five or six the amount of 'balancing' movements decreases and the ability to stand on one leg is similar for each side.

It should be noted that the leg of preference for standing and hopping is not always the same as the leg of preference for playing football, for instance. Asymmetrical performances should be interpreted very carefully; in extreme cases they may reflect a lateralisation syndrome, in which case there will undoubtedly be other signs of nervous dysfunction with an analogous pattern.

Involuntary movements, particularly choreiform movements or tremor, may strongly interfere with optimal performance. A low score for each leg, which is not accompanied by dyskinesia, may result from a retardation in functional maturation, generalised hypotonia, cerebellar or sensory dysfunction.

Hopping (Fig. 40)

Procedure

The child is asked to hop on each foot at least 20 times, starting with whichever leg he prefers. Hopping on the spot is preferable, but children younger than seven often cannot manage this and should be allowed to move forward.

Recording

The performance on each foot is recorded separately and the preferred leg noted.

    0 = unable to hop
    1 = 2-4 hops
    2 = 5-8 hops
    3 = 9-12 hops
    4 = 13-16 hops
    5 = 17-20 hops
    6 = more than 20 hops

Significance

The development of this motor function is also abrupt and rapid. At the age of three, only a few children are able to hop even a few times and then generally on one foot only; at four, 5-8 times is normal; at five, 9-12 times is possible; at six, 13-16 times is possible and about 25 per cent can already hop more than 20 times on one foot at least; at seven to eight years, the majority of children can hop more than 20 times with each foot.

Between the ages of five and seven, one leg is often better than the other one, though, as with standing on one leg, the best leg is not necessarily the preferred leg in playing football, for example. The relationship of hopping to the concept of dominance is a complex one. Consequently, an asymmetrical performance must be very carefully interpreted. The greater the discrepancy between left and right, the greater the possibility of a hemisyndrome or other lateralisation syndrome as the underlying cause. If such a lateralisation is present, other neurological findings should corroborate it.

A weak performance on both sides may reflect a retardation in maturation; neurogenic, myogenic, static or arthrogenic causes must also be considered. Pain from a different origin may also interfere with performance.

It is possible that training may influence results, but as most children at play hop only on their leg of preference, the training will be asymmetrical. As in the case of other tests such as diadochokinesis and standing on one leg, girls tend to perform better than boys.

CHAPTER 6

Assessment of the Trunk

Behavioural State

The optimal state of the child for the following series of tests is 0, though the tests are possible if it is 1.

Position

At this point in the examination, the child should undress to allow inspection of the trunk, and the elicitation of responses such as the abdominal skin and Galant responses. The child should stand relaxed, his feet equidistant from the midline, his head centred and his arms hanging by his side.

Age

These tests are suitable for all children aged 3 to 10.

Inspection of the Back
Procedure

The examiner should carefully inspect the spine and the skin of the back.

Recording

Any deviations from normal erect posture and any peculiarities of the skin are described. The movements of the spine forward, backward, to the side and in rotation are inspected and described if abnormal. Special attention should now be paid to possible lateral incurvation of the spine (*i.e.* scoliosis), particularly if observation of sitting, standing and walking has already aroused the suspicion of scoliosis.

Significance

Normally the thoracic part of the back is slightly curved forward while the lumbar part shows a certain degree of lordosis; there may be considerable variability between individuals (see Figs. 13-17, page 31). A lateral incurvation is always abnormal. In hypotonic children, thoracic kyphosis and lumbar lordosis may be accentuated.

The skin along the midline of the back is worth particularly careful inspection. Naevi, dimples, hairy patches or slight lipomas may be the only external signs of an underlying spina bifida occulta.

Naevi ordered laterally from the midline and often in dermatome areas (café-au-lait spots) or slight fibromas, etc., may arouse the suspicion of Recklinghausen's disease before the appearance of other symptoms. The naevi vasculosi which accompany Sturge-Weber's disease may be present on the skin of the back when they are not very conspicuous in the trigeminal area of the face; more often, they are not confined just to the skin of the back. Sebaceous adenomas may be a sign of tuberous sclerosis before the disease is clinically evident.

Any limitation of the movement of the spine should be further explored, especially if corroborated by findings during palpation. It may be of neurological or articular origin. In the case of scoliosis, a skeletal anomaly should be suspected but it may also result from unilateral hyper- or hypotonia, or unilateral irritating processes (see page 32).

SKIN REFLEXES

Abdominal Skin Reflex (Fig. 41)
Procedure

The examiner scratches with a pin from the side of the abdominal wall towards the centre, above, on a level with and below the navel.

Response

There should be a contraction of the abdominal muscles in the stimulated area.

Recording

     0 = absent
     1 = weak, just discernable reaction
     2 = marked contraction

Cremasteric Reflex (Figs. 42 and 43)
Procedure

The examiner takes a pin and scratches down the inner side of the upper leg.

Response

There should be a quick elevation of the testis; a bilateral response may be obtained.

Recording

     0 = absent
     1 = weak, barely discernable elevation of the testis
     2 = marked elevation of the testis

Galant Response (Fig. 44)
Procedure

The examiner takes a pin and scratches slowly along a paravertebral line about 5 cm from the midline from shoulder to buttock.

Response

The spine curves in with the concavity on the stimulated side. Only an immediate tonic response in one plane can be considered; other movements may occur as a result of tickling and cannot be interpreted as a Galant response.

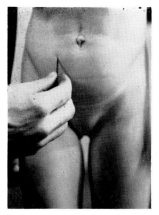
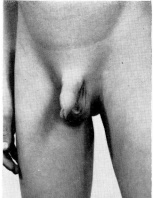
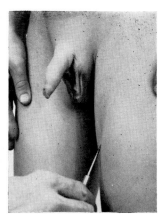

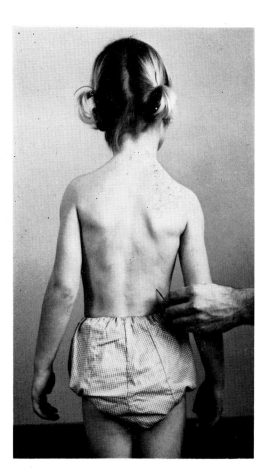

Above, left to right:

Fig. 41. Elicitation of the abdominal skin reflex in the right lower quadrant.

Fig. 42. Elicitation of the cremasteric reflex: position of the testicles before stimulation of the inner side of the upper leg.

Fig. 43. On scratching the inner side of the upper leg, the testicle on the same side is elevated.

Left:

Fig. 44. Elicitation of the Galant response on the right.

Recording

      0 = absent

      1 = barely discernable incurvation

      2 = marked incurvation

Significance

The Galant response may rarely be found in children younger than five, but is usually absent in older children. Absence of the abdominal skin reflex may be due to spinal dysfunction at specific levels; a supraspinal lesion may modify the excitability of the spinal centre of the reflex. However, depression or absence may well be due to non-neurological causes (*e.g.* acute surgical problem, distended bladder, surgical scarring of the skin, strong distension of the abdominal muscles caused by ascites). Absence of the cremasteric reflex may be due to non-neurological causes such as cold, nervousness, hydrocele or cryptotorchism.

The abdominal skin reflex and the cremasteric reflex should be symmetrical; asymmetries may be of significance if other lateralised signs in the same pattern occur.

The segmental levels for the abdominal skin reflex are Th.7-L1, for the Galant response Th.3-L1 and for the cremasteric reflex L1 and L2.

CHAPTER 7

Assessment of the Child Lying

Behavioural State

The optimal state of the child for the following series of tests is 0, though the tests are possible if it is 1 or 2.

Position

The child must lie prone on the examination table with his head centred and relaxed.

Age

These tests are suitable for all children aged 3 to 10, unless otherwise stated.

Examination of the Spine

Procedure

The examiner palpates the spinous processes, paying special attention to the lower lumbar and upper sacral vertebrae. As he does so, the child is asked to move his back sideways, to bend it and to hyperextend it. Particular attention should also be paid to the occurrence of scoliosis, especially if it was present when the child was standing.

Recording

Any abnormalities must be noted and described, including a missing spinous process or any limitation of movement.

Significance

A missing spinous process may indicate a spina bifida occulta and further X-ray analysis is necessary. Similarly, further exploration, *e.g.* X-rays, is necessary if there is any limitation of spinal movement. A scoliosis that persists in the lying position is generally caused by a skeletal abnormality.

Posture of the Legs and Feet

Procedure

The examiner looks for any asymmetries in the posture of the legs and feet, making sure that the child is lying straight with his legs relaxed; this can be confirmed by passively rotating the feet. After examination of the hip joint (see page 63), the child is asked to turn over so that an inspection can be carried out in the supine position.

Recording

An asymmetrical posture of legs and feet is described by scoring for abduction, adduction, flexion, extension, exorotation and endorotation respectively; the scores range from 0 to 2, 0 being the neutral position.

Significance

In hemisyndromes, an asymmetrical posture of the legs and feet in the lying position (prone or supine) may be present as the only postural manifestation. However, it must be stressed again that in most instances a single finding is of no clinical significance and must therefore be dealt with very cautiously.

Examination of the Hip Joints (Fig. 45)

Procedure

After inspection of the posture of the legs, the examiner stabilizes the child's pelvis with one hand and retroflexes the upper leg with the other hand. After the child has turned over into the supine position, the examiner flexes and extends the upper leg, and tests for abduction and adduction of the hip joint. By rotating the lower leg (with the knee bent), exo- and endorotation of the upper leg and the hip joint are tested.

Recording

The same criteria are applied as in the assessment of other joints (see 'Resistance against Passive Movements', page 14).

Significance

Asymmetrical findings at the hip joint may suggest a lateralisation, but orthopaedic causes must first be excluded.

It is essential that the pelvis be kept fixed so that movements of the pelvis do not camouflage limitation of movement by the hip.

Fig. 45. Examination of resistance to passive movements in the right hip. Flexion, abduction, adduction and rotation are tested with the child in the supine position.

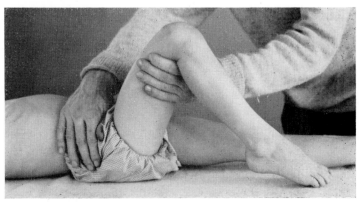

Knee-heel Test (Figs. 46 and 47)

Age

This test is suitable for children aged 6 to 10.

Procedure

The child is asked to lie on his back with his arms by his sides. He is then asked to put the heel of one foot on the knee of the other leg and to keep it there. After a few seconds, he is asked to move his heel down his leg towards the foot without losing contact with the leg. The test is repeated three times for each leg.

Response

All movements should be smooth and steady.

Recording

Accurate placing: 0 = accurate placing each time
                      1 = one or two errors of placement
                      2 = more than two errors of placement

Sliding heel down
    leg: 0 = smooth and steady, no slips
                      1 = one or two slips
                      2 = more than two slips; unable to keep heel in contact
                          with lower leg.

Fig. 46. The child closes her eyes and places one heel on the knee of the other leg.
Fig. 47. She moves her foot down her shin, keeping her eyes closed.

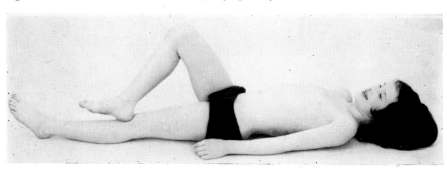

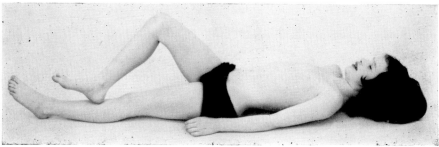

Significance

This is a useful test of coordination of the legs in which cerebellar and proprioceptive functions play a part. An asymmetrical performance related to dominance may be expected in six to seven-year-olds. In children over seven, asymmetry reflects an impairment of the coordination of one leg.

Sitting up without the Help of Hands (Figs. 48 and 49)

Procedure

Still lying on his back, the child is asked to sit up without supporting himself with his hands.

Recording

        0 = cannot sit up without support of hands
        1 = sits up without support of hands, but lifts legs.
        2 = sits up without support of hands, and without lifting legs.

When sitting up without support of the hands is accompanied by lifting of the legs, this must be recorded as symmetrical or asymmetrical and the latter described further.

Fig. 48. A seven-year-old child can sit up without the help of hands, keeping her legs in contact with the floor.

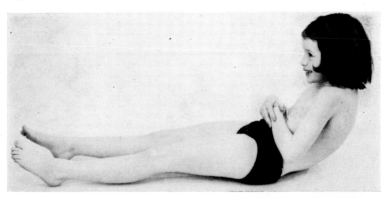

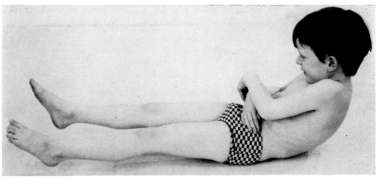

Fig. 49. A five-year-old can only sit up without the help of hands by lifting his legs from the floor.

65

Significance

Many children under the age of six may not be able to perform this test, and the examiner may assist by putting his hand under the child's head, while the child keeps his hands folded on his abdomen. Lifting of the legs may still be observed. Over the age of seven or eight, most children can sit up without lifting their legs. An asymmetrical lifting of the legs or a symmetrical exaggerated lifting may be due to cerebellar dysfunction.

At the end of this section of the examination, the child may get dressed again.

CHAPTER 8

Assessment of the Head

Behavioural State
   The optimal state of the child for the following series of tests is 0, though the tests are possible if it is 1.

Age
   These tests are suitable for all children aged 3 to 10.

Position
   The position of the child is not important. The assessment can be carried out with the child standing beside the sitting examiner. The head should be centred and symmetrical in relation to the body.

Musculature of the Face

Procedure
   The examiner must observe the facial musculature at rest and then during voluntary and emotional movements. For this purpose, the child is asked to show his teeth, frown, blow out his cheeks and then close his eyes. After the last instruction, the examiner presses in the child's cheeks and carefully tries to open his eyes. Emotional movements can be observed during laughing and crying.

Recording
   Facial musculature is scored three times for asymmetry: at rest, during voluntary movements and during emotional movements.
      0 = no asymmetry
      1 = slight asymmetry
      2 = marked asymmetry

Significance
   Unilateral peripheral facial palsies show an asymmetry in both upper and lower parts of the face, whereas a supranuclear lesion shows ipsilateral asymmetry, especially on the lower part of the face. In these cases, the aspect of the facial musculature during emotional movements may be relatively less affected. However, when a nuclear or peripheral lesion is involved the face is affected at all times.
   It is often difficult to assess the symmetry or asymmetry of the neuromuscular functioning of the facial musculature, as many children may have a somewhat asymmetrically shaped skull and face. It may occasionally be necessary to measure the distance between the lateral corner of the eye and the corner of the mouth on each

side of the face, and the distance between the ear and the corner of the mouth. It is always worth inspecting the child's head from above to detect any sign of plagiocephaly which might influence the symmetry of the face. From the age of four years, some children may develop habitual, often asymmetrical, features without any clear neurological significance.

EYES

Position (Fig. 50)

Procedure

The examiner must look for concomitant or non-concomitant strabismus. Slight squints may be detected by looking for symmetry of the corneal reflections. The 'cover test' may be used to detect latent strabismus or heterophoria: each eye is covered in turn while the child looks at a distant object (which does not require convergence). A slight movement may be observed in the uncovered eye either immediately after the other eye is covered or, more often, when the cover is removed. This test is based on the fact that in heterophoria, external eye muscle activity is needed to prevent diplopia, even when the eyes are 'resting'. When one eye is covered, this necessity disappears and the eye muscles can relax. As soon as the cover is removed, contraction of one or more of the eye muscles becomes necessary again, manifesting itself in a slight movement of the eye. The eye which shows movements is the eye with heterophoria.

Fig. 50. Position of the eyes for looking at a distance.

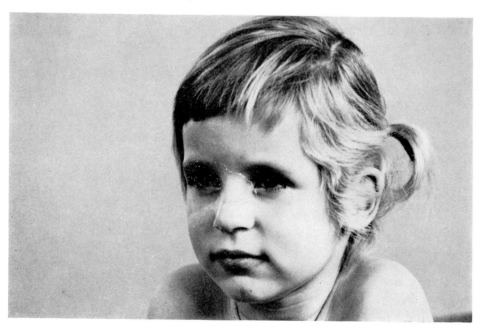

When the eye drifts towards the temporal side, the condition is known as exophoria; to the nasal side it is known as esophoria; upwards as hyperphoria and downwards as hypophoria.

If the eye muscles are not able to bring the visual axes to bear upon the same point, squint or strabismus is present (exotropia, esotropia, hypertropia or hypotropia respectively). In this event, the only way to avoid diplopia is to suppress one image, which leads to a reduction of visual acuity in the squinting eye.

Latent squint may also be observed during the tests for fixation (see below) and convergence (see page 71).

Recording

The presence or absence of heterophoria, concomitant strabismus or non-concomitant strabismus must be recorded. Where present, the eye involved and the type of heterophoria or squint must be described. In the case of non-concomitant strabismus, the eye muscles involved must be described by observing the movements the child is able to make when following an object in his visual field.

Significance

The detection of heterophoria is most important since its presence may hamper the child's ability in close work such as reading, drawing and writing, the muscular strain required leading to fatigue. An accurate estimate of visual acuity (see page 74) is an essential part of assessing how much the eye has deteriorated as a result of a manifest strabismus; in such a case, there is usually an impairment of visual acuity in one eye, especially in children aged five and over. However, amblyopia ex anopsia does not necessarily occur in children aged three or four, since these children often use both eyes alternately (*i.e.* alternate monocular vision).

In true concomitant strabismus, the angle between the two axes should remain constant over the entire range of eye-movements, though this is not invariably true. Concomitant strabismus may be due to optic, sensory, anatomic or nervous causes, but the cause is often unknown, especially in the case of congenital strabismus. A hereditary factor is often present, while it may also be found in children with a history of a birth trauma or short gestation.

Non-concomitant strabismus may result from oculo-paresis due to various causes (*e.g.* congenital or traumatic factors, disease of the orbita, intoxications, infectious diseases, diseases of the central nervous system or eye muscle diseases). Of particular interest is a generally benign and often transient paresis of the sixth cranial nerve some weeks after an otitis media or upper respiratory infection. A paresis of the ocular muscles of long standing may eventually result in a concomitant strabismus (Fig. 51).

Fixation

Procedure

The child is asked to fixate an object (such as the point of a pencil) which is held in front of his eyes for 15 seconds at a distance of about 40 cm. Three aspects are considered: deviation of one or both eyes; choreiform movements (*i.e.* jerky movements of both eyes which occur irregularly and arhythmically); and manifest strabismus.

69

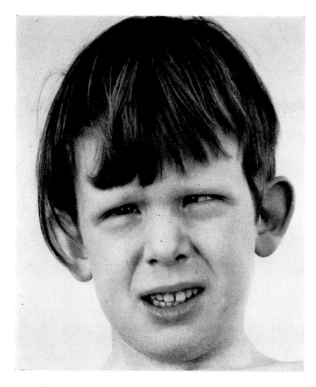

Fig. 51. Position of the eyes in a boy with a longstanding paresis of the sixth cranial nerve on the left side. The strabismus is concomitant.

Recording

Deviation, choreiform movements and squint are recorded as absent or present, and the involved eye and direction of the deviation or squint are specified.

Significance

Deviation of one eye during fixation may be due to a latent strabismus (heterophoria) or to an ocular paresis (see page 69). The significance of choreiform movements is discussed on page 76 and strabismus on page 69.

Visual Pursuit Movements

Procedure

The examiner moves a small object in front of the child in both the horizontal and the vertical plane. The child is asked to follow the object with his eyes, keeping his head still. Two aspects are assessed: the quality and the range of the ocular movements. Movements may be smooth, ataxic or choreiform. The last category is used for vertical jerky movements when the eyes move sideways and horizontal jerky movements when the eyes move upwards and downwards, occurring in both eyes simultaneously.

Recording

Abnormal following is described and any restriction of the full range of movements is recorded. Choreiform and ataxic eye movements are recorded as absent or

70

TABLE IV
Action of individual eye muscles

M. rectus lateralis:	to the temporal side
M. rectus medialis:	to the nasal side
M. rectus superior:	upwards and slightly inwards
M. rectus inferior:	downwards and slightly inwards
M. obliques superior:	downwards and slightly outwards
M. obliques inferior:	upwards and slightly outwards

present. During this test the examiner can also ascertain the presence of concomitant or non-concomitant strabismus, and in the latter case, which muscles are involved (see Table IV).

Significance

Deviations in the visual pursuit of an object may be due to paresis of the ocular muscles. Diplopia is rarely found in children because of rapid cortical suppression of one image. Ataxic movements may be due to impaired coordination of the eye muscles. The significance of choreiform movements is discussed on page 76.

Convergence (Fig. 52)
Procedure

An object is held at a distance of about 50 cm from the child and is moved towards him.

Fig. 52. Convergence of the eyes in looking at a close object. Compare with Fig. 51.

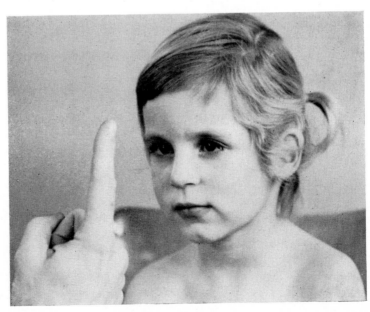

Response

The eyes converge on the object and the pupils contract.

Recording

>   0 = no convergence visible at all.
>   1 = unable to maintain convergence with the object closer than 12 cm to
>   the eyes.
>   2 = maintains convergence of both eyes on an object to about 7 cm in
>   front of the eyes.

Any differences in convergence between the eyes are recorded. Pupillary reaction is also recorded as absent or present.

Significance

Movements should be the same on both sides. A symmetrical weakness is generally of central origin; an asymmetrical weakness may be due to a paresis of an ocular muscle or to amblyopia of one eye. Weakness of convergence may also be caused by myopia or severe hypermetropia.

In cases of exophoria, convergence demands more muscle activity than usual and may therefore be rather weak; conversely, in cases of esophoria, convergence may be very strong.

Weakness of convergence may give rise to considerable difficulties as far as close work is concerned, leading to fatigue, etc.

Contraction of the pupils (miosis) during convergence is a sign of the accommodation of the lens, which is linked with the activity of the ciliary body. Absence of miosis may be due to the use of drugs, to a functional disturbance of the intraocular muscles, or to a mechanical cause.

Nystagmus

Nystagmus consists of involuntary oscillatory eye movements, usually with a slow and a rapid component. The latter is used to give the direction of the nystagmus.

Procedure

The examiner holds an object about 50 cm from the child and notes the occurrence of spontaneous nystagmus. The child is then asked to keep his head still while the examiner moves the object 45° sideways and to fixate on the object for about ten seconds in the new position. This is repeated at a 45° angle on the other side. A nystagmus occurring in these latter situations is called a directional nystagmus.

Recording

The presence or absence of spontaneous and directional nystagmus is recorded and the direction of the rapid component described if present. The intensity of the nystagmus should also be described and a note made of any asymmetries.

Significance

A horizontal, pendular nystagmus which is present from shortly after birth is called 'congenital nystagmus'. Its etiology is obscure; the intensity may be affected by the position of the head. Nearly always, vision is impaired. Spontaneous nystagmus may be due to disturbances of the vestibular system, which may be of infectious, toxic, traumatic or other origin.

In most cases, directional nystagmus is of vestibular origin but it may be due to a functional weakness of the eye muscles.

Optokinetic Nystagmus
Procedure

It is of little practical value, within the scope of this book, to introduce complicated techniques for the accurate evaluation of optokinetic nystagmus. However, it may be useful to know whether this nystagmus can be elicited laterally and vertically with the same frequency and intensity. For this purpose, it suffices to move a picture strip in front of the child's eyes in all four directions at a distance of about 40 cm. The child is instructed to try to follow these movements and is not intentionally prevented from doing so. Provided that the speed of movement of the strip is approximately the same in all directions, the optokinetic nystagmus elicited in this way should show the same frequency.

Recording

The presence or absence of horizontal and vertical optokinetic nystagmus is recorded and any asymmetry is noted. A difference in frequency between the eyes should also be recorded.

Significance

Horizontal optokinetic nystagmus should be elicitable in this way. Vertical optokinetic nystagmus is often more difficult to observe, especially when moving the strip downwards. A different frequency beween the two eyes is always pathological and should arouse the suspicion of an intracerebral lesion. Asymmetry of the optokinetic nystagmus in opposite directions may be of cerebral or peripheral origin, *e.g.* functional disturbances in the optical and/or vestibular systems.

A faulty response on this test may also be the consequence of diminished vision in one or both eyes.

Pupillary Reactions
Procedure

The size of the pupil is recorded and then a bright light is flashed into one eye only and the reactions of both pupils observed. This is repeated with the other eye. The child should be in such a position that light from outside or from a ceiling-light falls on both eyes equally.

Response

Pupillary reactions may be absent, slow or fast. If a light is thrown into one eye (direct reaction), the contralateral pupil (indirect reaction) should contract simultaneously with the stimulated pupil.

Recording

The size of the pupil is recorded as small, medium or large, and irregularities are described.

Direct pupillary reaction to light: 0 = absent
    1 = weak
    2 = strong

Indirect pupillary reaction to light: 0 = absent
    1 = weak
    2 = strong

Significance

Reaction to light should be prompt and marked. No contraction of the pupils may be due to peripheral or central causes. A negative indirect reaction results from unilateral blindness, caused by a lesion of the optic nerve. A weak and slow contraction may be due to drugs, infections, postinfectious conditions or a generalized depression of nervous functions.

Visual Acuity

Procedure

The examiner can test the older child's visual acuity by use of the Snellen Letter Charts. The Stycar tests can be used for children who cannot read letters (Sheridan 1969). This test, in which the child matches letters, makes it relatively easy to test visual acuity down to the age of three. These methods often give better results than the well known illiterate E-chart or picture chart.

Recording

Visual acuity is recorded as normal or abnormal, in which case a description is required.

Significance

The optimal 6/6 vision should not be expected before the age of six or seven; children younger than this are often hypermetropic. However, in cases of doubt, referral to an ophthalmologist for skiascopy is necessary (see page 1).

Visual Field (Figs. 53 and 54)

Procedure

The examiner sits down with the child standing in front of him so that their faces are on the same level. He asks the child to fixate on his nose (or a small object held about 40 cm. in front of the child). Then he moves a small object from one side of and from behind the child's head so that it gradually enters his visual field. The child is instructed to grasp the object as soon as he catches sight of it. The test is carried out from each side and from above the child's head. By sitting immediately in front of the child, the examiner is able to observe whether the child fixates well. A crude impression can thus be obtained about the child's visual fields. The test can

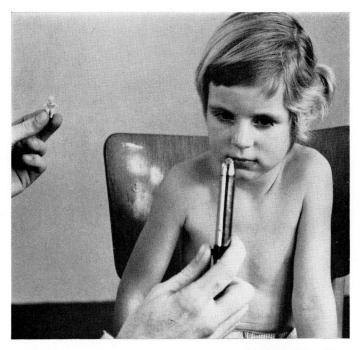

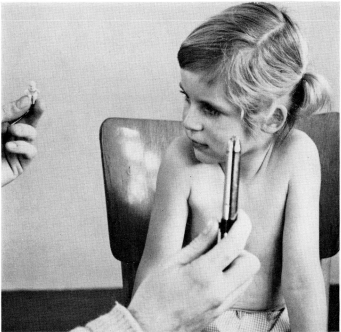

Fig. 53 (above). Position for the evaluation of the visual fields: the child looks at an object held in front of her while a toy is brought nearer from behind. **Fig. 54 (below).** The response.

be repeated with objects of different sizes and colours. Children aged over six may be asked to cover one eye with their hands or a wooden spoon.

Response

The normal angle of vision to the side is between 60° and 80° and above is about 45°.

Recording

The estimated angle at which the child perceives the object is recorded after each test and noted to be normal or abnormal.

Significance

The most common visual field defects in children are homonymous hemianopia, which generally accompanies spastic hemiplegia, and bitemporal hemianopia resulting from tumours near the optic chiasm, which may arise quite insidiously. Lesser defects, such as quadrantic defects of the visual fields, are rare (deriving from craniopharyngioma or a temporal lobe tumour involving the optic radiation.) Although such cases evidently surpass the bounds of minor dysfunction, a visual field defect may be the first clinical sign. The above test is sufficient for routine purposes, but if there is any doubt, perimetry should be carried out; however, this may be rather difficult and unreliable in children below the age of six or seven.

The examiner must bear in mind that diminished visual acuity may be responsible for diminished visual fields.

As with other tests of visuo-ocular abilities, any abnormal findings warrant referral to an ophthalmologist.

Choreiform Movements of the Face

Procedure

Throughout the examination of the eyes, the presence or absence of choreiform movements of the face should be assessed. There may be some difficulty in differentiating between choreiform movements and 'tics', especially in the upper part of the face, but the latter tend to show a more stereotyped pattern.

Recording

Choreiform movements are recorded as absent or present.

Significance

See pages 40 and 85.

Funduscopy

Funduscopy is carried out as the final assessment of the entire examination (see page 82), but may usefully be discussed here. It is not usually necessary to dilate the pupils pharmacologically for a routine inspection of the optic disc; however, in cases of doubt it may be necessary to use a mydriatic agent.

A discussion of all the different types of anomalies of the retina is beyond the scope of this book. For a routine screening it is sufficient to examine the fundus for papilledema, which may indicate increased intracranial pressure and in rare cases may be the first manifestation of an extensive intracranial lesion. When other anomalies of the retina are present, such as black spots, white streaks, vascular anomalies, etc., often a more specific examination must be carried out. It must be borne in mind that anomalies in refraction may considerably hamper inspection of the fundus.

EARS

Auditory Acuity
Procedure

The examiner sits about six yards away from the child and in a low voice pronounces test words of different sound spectra ('66', '100', '99') including single consonantal sounds ('sss', 'rrr', 'mmm') and vowel sounds ('uuuu', 'aaaa'). Each ear is tested in turn, the child keeping the other ear covered with his hand and repeating the sounds as heard. Children below the age of six may be asked to point to pictures; schemes suited to the English language have been devised by Sheridan (1969).

Recording

Auditory acuity in each ear is recorded as correct, dubious or failed.

    0 = correct
    1 = dubious
    2 = failed

Significance

A dubious response indicates the need for further audiological examination. It is of course highly desirable for pure tone audiometry to be carried out as a routine part of the examination, but the doctor should always screen hearing himself.

Localisation of Sound
Procedure

The examiner stands behind the child and gently rings a small bell on each side of his head and then above his head.

Response

The child is asked to point towards the place where the sound comes from. He is not expected to say 'left', 'right' or 'above', since this is not a test of his ability to comprehend and distinguish these concepts.

Recording

        0 = no localisation at all
        1 = localisation correct laterally
        2 = localisation correct in all directions

Significance

Most but not all children aged five and over are able to achieve accurate vertical localisation; this may be regarded as a maturational phenomenon. However, a negative response is of dubious significance in our present state of knowledge. Failure to locate sounds in any lateral position indicates the need for further audiological analysis.

MOUTH

Tongue

Procedure

The child is asked to stick out his tongue and keep it as still as possible. After about ten seconds, voluntary movements of discomfort may occur. Any occurrence of involuntary movements should be carefully noted, and then the child is asked to move his tongue from side to side, touching the corners of his mouth. Finally, he is asked to protrude it as far as possible.

Recording

Choreiform movements:	absent or present
Fasciculations:	absent or present
Smoothness of movements:	absent or present

Significance

A discussion of the significance of choreiform and athetoid movements can be found on pages 40 and 85.

Fasciculations are asynchronous, irregular, rapid twitches of very small parts of the tongue. The tongue is the only muscle in which they can be observed, myograms being necessary for other muscles. They must be differentiated from choreiform movements which occur in more extended areas of the tongue and lead to gross movements. Their significance is also different, since fasciculations are generally a sign of a serious, progressive disease (*e.g.* bulbar disorders).

Children over the age of seven or eight should be able to move their tongue smoothly from side to side and to protrude it for more than one third of its visible length. Awkwardness of tongue movements or a short frenum of the tongue is often related to speech disturbances.

Pharyngeal Arches

Procedure

The child is asked to open his mouth as wide as possible so that the examiner can inspect the pharyngeal arches at rest. Then the child is asked to say 'aaaa' so that the examiner may inspect them during movement.

Recording

The arches are recorded as symmetrical or asymmetrical and described in the latter instance.

Significance

Asymmetries of the pharyngeal arches, particularly during phonation, may be related to difficulties in speech and speech development. However, for several weeks or even months after tonsillectomy, some children may show temporary asymmetry of the movement of the arches, without evident impairment of speech or swallowing.

SPONTANEOUS MOTOR ACTIVITY

At this juncture, it is important for a reassessment of spontaneous motor activity to be made. Children with minor nervous dysfunction sometimes show a particularly marked increase or even a decrease in this field.

CHAPTER 9

General Data

When the assessment of the head has been concluded (except for funduscopy), the neurological examination is virtually completed. However, there are certain aspects of the general pediatric and developmental examination which may yield important information to the neurologist. For instance, the relationship of the child's weight to his height is relevant to an assessment of clumsiness, since an overweight child is likely to be more clumsy than a child of slender build. It is useful, therefore, to weigh and measure the child, and also to measure the circumference of the skull (for micro- or macrocephaly) and to describe any abnormalities in the shape of the skull (for plagiocephaly, synosteosis of a single suture, etc.). In clinical practice, abnormal findings as a result of the general pediatric examination with regard to the lungs and heart, the mucous membranes, ears and throat and general malformations may be significant and can usefully be recorded.

In practice, too, the examiner may wish to employ some of the tests of the type described in the Introduction (page v), which are not satisfactory in strict neurological terms, but which may yield valuable information if carefully interpreted. Such tests are often behavioural items which are also the appropriate sphere of the psychologist. Each examiner will develop his own preferences in this sort of testing, and objective data are lacking for guidance. The following may provide a useful outline.

Dominance

In a discussion of this problem, a careful distinction must be made between 'dominance', which we use to imply something about neurological organisation, suggesting that one hemisphere is superior to the other in controlling motor function, and 'preference' which describes the hand, foot or eye the child prefers to use for particular tasks.

Hand Preference

We use three tests of hand preference: drawing (which also serves for an assessment of fine motor coordination), writing, and cutting a piece of paper. The necessary implements are handed to the child in a neutral position, with no bias to right or left. Children over the age of five or six can also be asked to catch a ball (approximately 'n times in each hand), so that the most capable hand may be recorded.

Preference

'oot preference is more difficult to assess. A child may prefer one leg for kicking
other for standing on one leg, while older children are able to use both legs

alternately for kicking (and both hands for catching a ball) without demonstrating any particular preference. We have found that of a mixed sample of 150 five-year-olds, 28 per cent hopped more than 13 times on their left legs, and 39.5 per cent hopped more than 13 times on their right leg. Often, an accurate assessment of preference can be obtained by asking the child which is his 'best' leg.

Eye Preference

To assess eye preference, we ask the child to look with one eye through a short tube or a hole in a piece of paper, first with the examiner holding the tube and then holding it himself. Older children, again, may be able to use either eye at will. It is possible that hand preference in holding the tube may influence the choice of eye for looking. Clearly, refraction anomalies and other possible sources of difference in the visual capacities of the eyes must be excluded prior to the assessment.

Significance

Where preference is consistent, it would seem reasonable to talk of dominance. The age at which dominance is established is a matter for debate, as is the question of mixed laterality, but it appears that preferences as regards certain actions are well established by the age of three or four. Despite our lack of knowledge about the nature or dominance, it is important to record it, and to attempt to distinguish it from asymmetry due to neurological damage.

Fine Motor Coordination

It must be borne in mind that any impressions formed about the child's agility in tasks such as dressing, handling buttons or tying shoe-laces must not be considered as solid data measuring well-known neurological phenomena. Such activities are highly complex and depend on many often inextricably interwoven parameters. A recording of the child's manipulative abilities may be of some interest, however, and may also be observed during the assessment of hand preference, for example. Small objects should be picked up in a 'pincer grasp', (*i.e.* opposition of the tips of the thumb and the index finger); long and narrow objects like a pencil, however, are often picked up with the thumb in opposition to three or four fingers. Children of five years and more should be able to hold the pencil between the thumb and index finger, whereas younger children often hold it between the second and third finger, and very young or severely retarded children may use the whole hand for drawing. However, observation of drawing does not generally add any clear information about neurological functions which cannot be obtained by more standardised neurological means.

Sensory Examination

As stressed in the Introduction, specific use of classical neurological tests such as two-point discrimination, tactile sensation with cotton wool, or pain and temperature perception have not proved particularly useful. Nevertheless, during the routine examination it is possible to make some general observations about the child's sensory functions. At some point in the examination the examiner can touch the child with a cold metal object and note his reaction and comments, if any. He can also record whether the child is sensitive to light touch and to the pin used in testing for the abdominal skin, Galant and cremasteric reflexes. Where there is any cause for doubt as to a child's sensitivity to tactile sensations, pain or differences in temperature, a more extensive examination should be carried out, but, as yet, no reliable methods of examination have been devised, particularly for children with learning and/or behavioural difficulties.

In older children, kinesthesia and sense of position in the thumbs and big toes can be tested by gently moving a thumb or toe and asking the child if he is aware of the movement. The child should keep his eyes closed during the test. He can then be asked to describe the position in which the examiner is holding the thumb or toe.

Speech and Language

As mentioned in the Introduction, there may be a close association between neurological dysfunction and speech disorders. Data obtained from an assessment of speech will clearly be relevant to the final assessment of the child with neurological dysfunction. It is usually possible to elicit sufficient speech from the child during the course of the 30 to 40 minute routine examination to decide whether a further intensive speech examination should form part of the assessment of each particular child. The examiner may observe many infantile speech faults such as substitutions, inversion, or perseverations during the neurological assessment, and he should hear enough speech to suspect that the child has difficulties or to decide that the child's use of language is appropriate to his age. It is a good idea to have toys and pictures in the examination room and to ask the child to name them.

If a child does not talk enough for an assessment to be made, the examiner should consult with psychological colleagues carrying out a behavioural assessment of the child. This is particularly important if the child has not spoken well. If the psychologist has also noted difficulties, speech and language specialists should commonly be called in to consultation. If there is any suspicion of dysarthria, a close examination of the mouth, tongue and palate is clearly important, and additional tests, probably with the aid of an ear, nose and throat specialist and a speech therapist may have to be carried out.

All these functions are recorded as indicated on the proforma (see page 102), and funduscopy can then be carried out as described in chapter 8.

CHAPTER 10

Interpretation and Diagnosis

The neurological examination must clearly be followed by an interpretation of findings. In most of the conditions with which this book is concerned, a final diagnosis will not be possible. Our method is to group together signs and symptoms in an attempt to identify specific diagnostic entities, which we refer to as syndromes. Other information apart from the findings of the neurological examination must be taken into consideration for a diagnosis to be made, *e.g.* causative patho-anatomical information, the natural history and the prognosis of the disease process.

The child's full history is naturally of primary importance, and should be obtained from the child's mother, preferably at the end of the examination. In this way, the examiner can avoid any bias which may influence findings, particularly when he is looking for only minor deviations in optimal functioning. In some rare cases, however, the history may allow a definite diagnosis to be made or suspected, *e.g.* a history of measles-encephalitis. A young child who has been referred to a clinic because of behaviour and/or learning difficulties may require a number of specialist assessments (pediatric, psychological, audiological, ophthalmological, speech, etc.) which must all be taken into account in an attempt to reach a final diagnosis. However, it is very important that some conclusion about the child's functioning should be drawn based on the findings of each particular assessment alone; the different examinations must therefore be carried out quite independently of each other.

This book is especially concerned with the conclusions that may be drawn from neurological signs, *i.e.* the way they tend to cluster, with the aim of describing syndromes. As we have emphasised throughout the book, a single non-optimal finding such as an isolated dorsoflexion of the big toe or an isolated exaggerated patellar tendon reflex is very rarely of clinical significance. When non-optimal signs are found in combinations, however, a valuable clinical interpretation may be made. Thus we aim to collect all non-optimal signs, order them into syndromes when this is possible, and then attempt to relate them by further study to other diagnostic information. Some such associations have already been established: we know that there is a close link between hyperexcitability in the newborn period (itself linked to obstetrical hazards) and the later appearance of certain distinct types of dyskinetic movement (see page 85); similarly, hemisyndromes in the newborn period are closely related to hemisyndromes at a later age.

We feel that a distinction between children with obvious neurological dysfunction and children with inconspicuous nervous dysfunction is a helpful one. By 'obvious', we mean cases which are easily identifiable before examination, such as a 'classic' case of cerebral palsy which can be identified as soon as the child walks into the room.

By 'inconspicuous', we mean cases of the type which are revealed only after the full neurological examination as described.

There is no clear-cut direct relationship between the degree of neurological dysfunction and the extent of behavioural disturbances. A child with an inconspicuous neurological disease may show as many or more disorganized patterns of behaviour as the child with a more obvious dysfunction. Society generally does not recognise his handicap and he is likely to receive less compensation and tolerance from his environment than the child with a recognised handicap; this may have important consequences for his overt behaviour.

In a very few cases, it may be possible to conclude specific behavioural disturbances to be the result of specific nervous dysfunctions, *e.g.* slight difficulties in co-ordination will involve clumsy behaviour. In most cases such a specific relation is not present. Therefore, it is clearly important to consider the coexistence in the same individual of a cluster of neurological signs and behavioural problems, which may range from specific problems of manipulation to problems of social relationships. We believe that it is important to assess the neurological parameter in any child who has behavioural and/or learning difficulties, but it should not be assumed that the coexistence of neurological and behavioural problems implies a common etiology. As far as we know, no valid correlations have been established between the neurological syndromes that we are about to describe and any specific types of behavioural problems. When we detect signs of neurological dysfunction in a child, our practice is to inform those responsible for his care and management (usually parents and teachers) that those abnormalities have been detected, but that we do not know what relationship they bear to the difficulties which brought the child to our attention. Thus, the possibility of a relationship is neither confirmed nor denied, while the child may benefit from the increased understanding of those around him.

We shall now discuss the various entities which may be distinguished from the ways in which isolated neurological signs tend to cluster. There may well exist considerable overlap between the groups while, on the other hand, a number of distinct signs of nervous dysfunction may be found which do not seem to hang together at all.

Hemisyndrome

By the terms 'hemisyndrome' or 'lateralisation syndrome', we mean a combination of neurological signs that together form a specific unilateral pattern. It should not be inferred that major functional difficulties are also present; by definition, all hemiplegias fall into the group of hemisyndromes, but a child with a hemisyndrome need not be hemiparetic. For instance, a hemisyndrome may consist of a combination of slightly increased (or decreased) tendon reflexes, slightly increased resistance to passive movements, a dorsiflexion of the big toe and some pronation of one of the extended arms, all on the same side of the body; from a superficial observation of the free-moving child, however, these may be quite inconspicuous. On the other hand, a hemisyndrome may consist of a paretic arm and leg of central origin, or of a unilateral peripheral nerve lesion.

Clearly, the signs which indicate a hemisyndrome may range from the very severe to the very mild. The mild forms do not generally interfere with ordinary everyday activities; fine motor coordination may be slightly impaired, but this is not necessarily the case.

The topographical and functional correlation of the different signs will facilitate a differentiation between their central or peripheral origin. As in the case of severe manifestations of hemisyndromes, mild forms may originate from pre- or paranatal brain damage, or may be acquired in infancy or childhood (due to trauma, infections, etc.). It must be borne in mind that mild signs of a hemisyndrome may be the first clinical manifestation of a progressive disorder such as a cerebral tumour, metabolic disorders or leucodystrophies.

Dyskinesia

Dyskinesia may occur in various forms, such as choreo-athetosis, chorea, athetoid cerebral palsy and dystonias, as well as choreiform movements, athetotiform movements, tremor and tics.

In choreo-athetosis, the lesion is situated in the striatum and basal ganglia, often due to kernicterus. It may be manifest in very severe or very mild form. Children with blood-group incompatibilities who underwent transfusions to prevent kernicterus may well show only very minor signs.

Huntingdon's chorea and other rare hereditary forms of chorea initially present with minor signs of dyskinesia. Chorea minor (Sydenham's chorea) which is caused by streptococcal infection may manifest itself in a very mild form, or may present with only mild choreatic movements as a sequela of the acute form.

Athetotiform and choreiform dyskinesias also range from very mild to severe. As mentioned previously (page 39), these terms are derived from the initial likeness to mild forms of athetosis and chorea. The movements are probably due to an instability of motor-units. This instability may take the form of a lowered membrane-potential of the motor cell itself, or may be related to changes in the excitatory and/or inhibitory input to the motor cell from other nerve cells. These neurophysiological changes may occur without a topographically circumscribed lesion of the brain.

Thus, choreiform movements may be considered as a noise phenomenon in a complex central system, the effect on motor functioning depending on the signal-noise ratio during a given performance. In very delicate motor activity, any non-relevant activity will interfere considerably, while in gross motor activity, the effect will be relatively less because of the higher rate of redundancy; this, at least, is the hypothesis which might explain such clearly demonstrable phenomena. A significant relationship has been found between the hyperexcitability syndrome in the neonatal period and the occurrence of choreiform movements in later life (Prechtl 1965). The etiology of choreiform movements has not yet been fully explained, but it is evident that pre- and paranatal complications as well as complications occurring in the first years of life such as severe respiratory diseases, gastrointestinal disturbances or head traumas play some part. A genetic factor may also be involved. It has been shown that the incidence of choreiform movements is two to three times higher in boys (Stemmer 1964).

Athetotiform movements are fairly frequent in children below the age of five to six years. Preliminary data suggest that they occur more frequently among special school pupils than among children attending ordinary primary schools, and that they are closely related to the presence of choreiform movements. The etiology of athetotiform movements is still obscure. The fact that some children show this type of movement while others do not, and that the movements decrease in intensity and frequency with age, suggest that they are a worthy topic of consideration in relation to minor nervous dysfunction.

A mild degree of resting tremor is often present in school children and characteristically does not interfere with even very fine manipulations, except in some rare instances. However, marked tremor does interfere considerably with fine motor activities. Tremor may occur in any muscle of the body, but it is usually most marked in the arms and fingers.

Associated Movements

Associated movements (known variously as synkinetic movements, co-movements, and mirror movements) often accompany voluntary or involuntary movements in young children, generally in contralateral and symmetrical parts of the body. They decrease with age, and their disappearance is reckoned to be a sign of the functional maturation of the nervous system. Several authors have emphasised the possibility of using the occurrence of associated movements over a certain age (which must be specified for each type of movement separately) as a sign of impaired neurological functioning, *i.e.* retardation of the nervous development (Abercrombie *et al.* 1964, Connolly and Stratton 1968, Fog and Fog 1963, Zazzo 1960). These authors have devised special tests for associated movements, but in our experience these tests are time-consuming and we prefer to assess associated movements at the same time as we test other aspects of the nervous system, *e.g.* diadochokinesis, walking on tiptoe and walking on heels.

The mouth-opening finger-spreading test does specifically test for associated movements, but the results should not be taken as a sound indication of the occurrence of associated movements in general, nor should the scoring be immediately related to the results of the tests advocated by other authors. As far as is known at the present, there is no direct relationship between the score on the mouth-opening finger-spreading test and the amount of associated movements occuring with diadochokinesis, walking on tiptoe or walking on heels. Preliminary observations suggest that there is not even any direct relationship between the amount of associated movements in the contralateral arm during the test for diadochokinesis and the amount of associated movements during clenching the fist, and this must be borne in mind when attempting to evaluate the occurrence of associated movements. Many factors may influence the amount of associated movements shown, *e.g.* the complexity of the movement involved, the intensity with which the 'trigger' movement is carried out, the order in which the tasks are presented and the familiarity with the requested 'trigger' movement. Many adults who do not show any associated movements when carrying out the test for diadochokinesis with the preferred hand do show them when carrying out the test with the non-preferred hand, especially if they do the test forcefully. Associated movements may also be seen in the tongue during writing. It does not need to be emphasised that the persistence of marked associated movements may interfere with many other acts.

Associated movements are often more marked on one side of the body and are probably related to cerebral dominance, the movements spreading to one side of the body more easily than to the other. It is not always easy to predict which side will be more affected. In older children, whose cerebral dominance is definitely established, spreading will generally occur from the non-dominant towards the dominant side, and this may be the normal or optimal situation. However, this is not true of all children. Two factors may be involved in these cases:—one is the wide variability in the age at which cerebral dominance is established, and the other is the fact that, in many individuals, dominance may not be strictly unilateral. Crossed laterality may occur not only between hands and feet, but in other forms of mixed laterality which are very difficult to demonstrate. Furthermore, the order in which the tests are applied and the skill on the side which has to perform the trigger movements may be of considerable importance in a comparison of associated movements on the left and right side of the body.

It is also possible that a strong asymmetry of associated movements may be part of a hemisyndrome, the neurologically impaired side showing more such movements. A high amount of associated movements may be found in combination with other signs of non-optimal nervous functioning, *e.g.* dyskinesias, co-ordination difficulties and evidence of hemisyndromes, etc. They may also be found in combination with other signs of motor retardation, such as an inability to continue hopping or standing on one leg for a sufficient amount of time or inadequate diadochokinesia, but without specific sign of nervous impairment. In the first instance, there may or may not be some developmental retardation, but clearly signs of nervous dysfunction play a dominant role; in the second instance, the developmental lag is the main or even the only feature of the child's neurological functioning. This differentiation is very important, since in the case of nervous dysfunction, the possibility of specific disorders, even progressive ones, must be considered, while developmental retardation may require a very different therapeutic approach.

Developmental Retardation

This term is generally used to include specific signs of mental retardation together with failure to develop certain behavioural skills such as building a tower with ten bricks, drawing a circle inside a square and speaking sentences of a given length at various specific ages. These problems may or may not be associated with neurological retardation. In the context of this book, developmental retardation means only a maturational lag in neurological functions such as walking, hopping, standing on one leg, diadochokinesia or the persistence of infantile reflexes, etc. The importance of the role of cerebral dominance in these instances has already been pointed out. Other signs of nervous dysfunction such as dyskinesia, a hemisyndrome or coordination difficulties may or may not be present. The possible combination of neurological retardation with mental retardation goes beyond the scope of this book, but it should be borne in mind that the two are not necessarily related.

The importance of an accurate differentiation between signs of neurological retardation that are accompanied by other signs of nervous dysfunction and those that are not has already been stressed (see above). However, developmental retardation may originate in nervous dysfunction due to cerebral damage while few other signs of this dysfunction are evident.

Difficulties in Coordination

Here again, it is essential to distinguish between impaired coordination and a retardation of coordination capabilities. This distinction may be very difficult or even impossible; the existence of other signs of neurological developmental retardation or, alternatively, signs of neurological dysfunction which are not due to developmental retardation may be helpful.

Several aspects of coordination may be distinguished, *e.g.* the maintenance of balance, the ability to anticipate shifts in the centre of gravity before making voluntary movements, the coordination of rapid rhythmical movements and of fine manipulations, and complex skilled motor performances. The brain structures involved are the proprioceptive system, including the vestibuli, the reticular formation and the cerebellum, and, in the case of complex motor behaviour, the parietal lobes.

The major complaint accompanying cases of mild disabilities of motor coordination is clumsiness and awkwardness. Fine motor coordination and gross motor coordination are not necessarily impaired simultaneously and to the same degree. The maturation of normal coordination is slow and much training and learning is involved. Walking without support, for instance, usually develops several months after the child can walk holding his mother's hands. A steady gait develops later still, after the acquisition of skilled balance. Fine manipulations such as doing up and undoing buttons should be possible at the age of four and tying up shoe-laces at the age of six. Diadochokinesia should be smooth and rapid by the age of eight.

Difficulties in coordination may be due to maturational retardation, defects in the proprioceptive system, parietal lobe dysfunction, intoxication, etc. Ingram (1967) has emphasised the incidence of hypoglaemic attacks in infancy and childhood as an often overlooked cause of slight coordination difficulties. The initial signs of progressive diseases may be slight disturbances of coordination such as difficulties in swallowing, articulation defects, unsteady gait or slight ataxia. This may be the case with cerebellar or brain stem tumours, metabolic disorders such as Hartnup disease, degenerative diseases (Friedrich's ataxia, ataxia teleangiectasia) and even disseminated sclerosis (Aigner and Siekert 1959).

Sensory Disturbances

It is well known that disturbances of vision or hearing, whether major or minor, may have profound effects on the child's learning capacities, and in recent years emphasis has been laid on the importance of detecting such defects at an early age. Slight abnormalities may remain undetected for a long time. For instance, partial deafness in which most of the sound spectrum is adequately perceived but a small part is missing may escape the attention of parents and teachers, and may result in the loss of important information for the child. Doctors should be alert to these possibilities.

The role of other disturbances of sensation is much less clear. In the more severely brain-damaged children, the whole field of visual perception disorders has been extensively studied (see, for example, Abercrombie's review 1964). Often it has not proved possible to distinguish between central problems of perception and the role of sensory loss itself. We ourselves, as mentioned previously, have found it difficult to devise adequate tests for sensory functioning, and can add little to a discussion of this topic. Minor disturbances such as slight defects in exteroceptive and proprioceptive perception may result in distorted pattern-formation in the brain. In cases of brain damage, auditory-visual interpretation and the ability to translate tactile and kinesthetic sensations into visual information, which normally develop between the ages of five and ten years, have been found to be defective (Belmont *et al.* 1966, Birch and Belmont 1965/1966, Birch and Bortner 1967).

Miscellaneous Signs (a Syndrome consisting of the Absence of a Syndrome)

It is evident that a considerable amount of overlap exists between the groups of signs which have been discussed so far. Indeed, it would be quite exceptional to find indications of one of these conditions without any signs that could not also belong to another group.

However, one may be confronted by a set of findings which do not show any clear relationship with one another, and from which no specific or recognisable pattern emerges. Such signs may be unequivocably and persistently present. For example, a child may show increased tendon reflexes on one side of the body, but an increased amount of associated movements on the other side, persistent infantile reflexes on the side of the increased tendon reflexes but alterations of the footsole reflex on the other side again, dominance may be very poorly expressed, and motor functions like hopping, kicking or fine finger manipulations may appear to be impaired on one or other side of the body, more or less at random.

Another example is the child who cannot tie up his shoe-laces, cannot cope with buttons, cannot ride a bicycle, etc., *i.e.* a child who shows many insufficiencies in motor behaviour, while few marked signs of nervous dysfunction are revealed by a strict neurological examination. Walton (1963) called such children 'clumsy children' and reported very few signs of nervous dysfunction which we have discussed on neurological examination; Illingworth (1963) reported marked signs which, however, did not show the same pattern in cases with the same deficits in motor functioning.

Clearly, the opposite pattern may also be found, *i.e.* children without any motor difficulties at all may still show marked signs of nervous dysfunction which cannot be arranged into specific patterns.

CHAPTER 11

The Relationship between Neurological Dysfunction and Behaviour

The nervous system must be considered as the apparatus for the performance of complex behaviour. A strict distinction between neurological phenomena as described in the previous paragraphs and certain aspects of behaviour, such as vigilance, attention span, persistence of visual fixation or voluntary goal-directed movements, is in fact purely artificial, and based only on the traditional distinction between neurology and psychology.

The different methodological basis for each discipline has led to a divergence in approach, while at the same time, the two modes of approach have often been mixed up, giving rise to much confusion. This is the case in the so-called syndrome of 'minor brain dysfunction'. Many studies carried out in this area suffer from serious methodological shortcomings, often combined with a wide acceptance of various superstitions, especially on the part of clinicians, while factual data are extremely limited.

In a group of children with behavioural and/or learning disorders or difficulties, some may show marked signs of nervous dysfunction when properly examined, while others showing similar behavioural disturbances will not. However, when a group of children exhibit both neurological and behavioural signs in common, a causal relationship may sometimes logically be inferred between the signs of nervous dysfunction and part of the behaviour exhibited. A patient with slight ataxia may show impairment of all behaviour patterns which require fine motor manipulation; thus he will be handicapped in his everyday behaviour. Each child will react to this sort of handicap in an individual manner, depending on a number of other variables. A child with marked choreiform jerks in the eye muscles may appear to have deficits in those behavioural patterns which require steady fixation, but the degree of handicap will depend on many other factors. Paroxysmal epileptic activity in the brain leading to a cessation of function will interrupt continuous performances, but in such cases, also, other factors determine the final behaviour of the child in his attempts to compensate for his handicap.

On the other hand, a logical relationship between signs of neurological dysfunction and the behavioural disturbances shown can more often not be implied. It is difficult to see how an asymmetrical abdominal skin reflex, a slight difference in the resistance against passive movements or slight asymmetry in the intensity of the tendon reflexes may lead to specific disturbed behaviour. Any conclusion as to a direct relationship would be premature, to say the least.

It must also be borne in mind that behaviour is influenced by many other factors of non-neurological origin. Together with genetical and exogenuous determinants, psychogenic and somatic conditions play a decisive role as regards overt behaviour. This complex cohesion of different factors makes any analysis of the relationship between neurological dysfunction and behavioural phenomena extremely difficult. The context of this book does not allow an extensive discussion of these factors, but their significance must not be overlooked and cannot be overestimated. However, a few points may be stressed. A nervous dysfunction which manifests itself in a child's behaviour will lead to reactive behaviour from his environment. This is true even at a very young age (Bell 1969, Prechtl 1963). For instance, the presence of signs of the hyperexcitability syndrome in the first few weeks of life may endanger the development of the child-mother interaction, involving uncertainty on the part of the mother which may persist throughout the years of the child's development and influence her relationship with the child as it grows up (Hart de Ruyter 1961).

Slight nervous dysfunction may sometimes hinder a child in his school work, though quite unspecifically, and his achievement will fall below the expectations of his parents or teachers. Repercussions of this may influence the parent-child relationship or the relationship between the child and the teacher. The resulting attitudes of parents, teachers and even playmates may inflict a burden on the child. Children with slightly less than optimal functioning of the nervous system seem particularly vulnerable to such environmental influences, so that a relationship between neurological dysfunction and behavioural disturbance may develop by this devious route.

Nevertheless, the same behavioural disturbances may exist without signs of nervous dysfunction. It must now be clear that in such cases a conclusion as to the existence of a syndrome of 'minor brain damage' is quite inadmissible.

Much basic research remains to be done. In connection with our interpretation of many findings of the neurological examination, our knowledge about normal nervous functioning is still remarkably small. For instance, a further validation of the maturation of abilities such as diadochokinesia, fine finger manipulations, tests of coordination, hopping, standing on one leg, etc., is badly needed. This applies, too, to the role of cerebral dominance in such functions, the development of hand and foot preference, the significance of dominance with regard to the presence of associated movements, and its maturational course.

In summary, one is forced to conclude that it is not possible to think in terms of simple relationships between disturbances of nervous functioning and of behaviour. In each child, it is necessary to evaluate separately the dynamics of the different factors that contribute to the establishment of his ultimate behaviour. There is a stringent need for data about all these different factors which must be collected without contamination from other sources. Perhaps it will then be possible to find a specific relationship between several of them, bearing in mind that in each individual the relationship may develop along different lines.

Examination Proforma for Minor Neurological Dysfunction

'State' and 'Social Responsiveness' are scored at each stage of the examination and any change in either should be scored in the column opposite the test in which the change occurred.

Unless otherwise indicated, the scoring on the left side of the proforma applies to the left side of the body, and that on the right to the right side of the body.

ASSESSMENT OF SITTING

									State	Soc. Resp.
Posture										
Head	0	1	2	rotated	0	1	2			
	0	1	2	bent laterally	0	1	2			
(ante)	0	1	2	flexion	0	1	2 (retro)			
Trunk	0	1	2	rotated	0	1	2			
	0	1	2	bent laterally	0	1	2			
	0	1	2	kyphosis	0	1	2			
	0	1	2	lordosis	0	1	2			
		symmetrically collapsed			0	1	2			
Legs	0	1	2	endorotation	0	1	2			
	0	1	2	exorotation	0	1	2			
	0	1	2	flexion	0	1	2			
	0	1	2	extension	0	1	2			
	0	1	2	adduction	0	1	2			
	0	1	2	abduction	0	1	2			
Feet	0	1	2	endorotation	0	1	2			
	0	1	2	exorotation	0	1	2			
	0	1	2	dorsiflexion	0	1	2			
	0	1	2	plantar flexion	0	1	2			
	0	1	2	adduction	0	1	2			
	0	1	2	abduction	0	1	2			
Spontaneous Motility										
Quantity		gross movements			0	1	2	3		
		small movements			0	1	2	3		
Quality		speed			0	1	2	3		
		smoothness			0	1	2	3		
		adequacy			0	1	2	3		
Involuntary Movements										
		absent								
		present (describe)								
Kicking										
0	1	2	3	median	0	1	2	3		
0	1	2	3	45° inwards	0	1	2	3		
0	1	2	3	45° outwards	0	1	2	3		
				total score						

EXAMINATION OF THE MOTOR SYSTEM

		State	Soc. Resp.

Muscle Power

0	1	2	3	neck	0	1	2	3
0	1	2	3	shoulders	0	1	2	3
0	1	2	3	elbows	0	1	2	3
0	1	2	3	wrists	0	1	2	3
0	1	2	3	hands	0	1	2	3
0	1	2	3	hips*	0	1	2	3
0	1	2	3	knees	0	1	2	3
0	1	2	3	ankles	0	1	2	3
0	1	2	3	feet	0	1	2	3

Resistance to Passive Movements

0	1	2	3	neck	0	1	2	3
0	1	2	3	shoulders	0	1	2	3
0	1	2	3	elbows	0	1	2	3
0	1	2	3	wrists	0	1	2	3
0	1	2	3	hands	0	1	2	3
0	1	2	3	hips*	0	1	2	3
0	1	2	3	knees	0	1	2	3
0	1	2	3	ankles	0	1	2	3
0	1	2	3	feet	0	1	2	3

Range of Movements**

Head   anteflexion
            retroflexion
            rotation
Shoulder abduction
            circumduction of arm
Elbow   extension
            flexion

Wrists   hyper-extension
            flexion
Hips   abduction
            circumduction of leg
Knees   extension
            flexion
Ankles   dorsiflexion
            plantar flexion
            rotation

*For practical reasons the results of the examination of the hips are recorded here, although the examination itself is carried out at a later stage of the procedure.
**Deviations from the average range of movements described in the text should be recorded as quantitatively as possible.

EXAMINATION OF REFLEXES

						State	Soc. Resp.
0 1 2 3 4	ankle jerk	0 1 2 3 4					
0 1 2 3	threshold	0 1 2 3					
0 1 2 3 4	knee jerk	0 1 2 3 4					
0 1 2 3	threshold	0 1 2 3					
0 1 2 3	biceps reflex	0 1 2 3					
0 1 2 3	threshold	0 1 2 3					
0 1 2 3	triceps reflex	0 1 2 3					
0 1 2 3	threshold	0 1 2 3					

Plantar Response

Big Toe 0 1 2 dorsiflexion 0 1 2
       0 1 2 plantar flexion 0 1 2

Other Toes 0 1 fanning 0 1
       0 1 2 plantar grasp 0 1 2

       0 1 2 3 palmo-mental reflex 0 1 2 3

ASSESSMENT OF STANDING

State   Soc. Resp.

Posture

Head
0 1 2 rotated 0 1 2
0 1 2 bent laterally 0 1 2
(ante) 0 1 2 flexion 0 1 2 (retro)

Trunk
0 1 2 rotated 0 1 2
0 1 2 bent laterally 0 1 2
0 1 2 kyphosis 0 1 2
0 1 2 lordosis 0 1 2
symmetrically collapsed 0 1 2
left shoulder lower than right: no, yes cm.
right shoulder lower than left: no, yes cm.

Upper Limbs
0 1 2 endorotation 0 1 2
0 1 2 exorotation 0 1 2
0 1 2 flexion 0 1 2
0 1 2 extension 0 1 2
0 1 2 adduction 0 1 2
0 1 2 abduction 0 1 2

Pelvis
left crista iliaca lower than right: no, yes cm.
right crista iliaca lower than left: no, yes cm.

Legs
0 1 2 endorotation 0 1 2
0 1 2 exorotation 0 1 2
0 1 2 flexion 0 1 2
0 1 2 extension 0 1 2
0 1 2 adduction 0 1 2
0 1 2 abduction 0 1 2

Feet   0   1   2   endorotation   0   1   2
          0   1   2   exorotation   0   1   2
          0   1   2   flexion   0   1   2
          0   1   2   extension   0   1   2
          0   1   2   adduction   0   1   2
          0   1   2   abduction   0   1   2

Arch of the Foot   left   cm. (without correction of
                                                        ankle position)
                            right   cm.
                            left   cm. (after correction of
                                                        ankle position)
                            right   cm.

                  pes planus:
                  pes excavatus:
                  distance between feet for balance:

Spontaneous Motility

Quantity   gross movements   0   1   2   3
              small movements   0   1   2   3
Quality   speed   0   1   2   3
              smoothness   0   1   2   3
              adequacy   0   1   2   3

Involuntary Movements
          absent
          present (describe)

Pronation of Arms (20″)
          0   1   2   spooning   0   1   2
          0   1   2   deviation from   0   1   2
                          median line
          0   deviation from   0
                          horizontal

Supination of Arms (20″)
          0   1   2   pronation   0   1   2

TESTS FOR INVOLUNTARY MOVEMENTS (20″)

      0   1   2   3   distal choreiform   0   1   2   3
                          movements
      0   1   2   3   proximal choreiform   0   1   2   3
                          movements
      0   1   2   3   athetotiform   0   1   2   3
                          movements
      0   1   2   3   choreatic movements   0   1   2   3
      0   1   2   3   athetotic movements   0   1   2   3
      0   1   2   3   tremor   0   1   2   3

State	*Soc. Resp.*

State	*Soc. Resp.*

TESTS FOR COORDINATION AND ASSOCIATED MOVEMENTS

						State	Soc. Resp.

0 1 2 3   mouth-opening finger-   0 1 2 3
           spreading
           phenomenon

   0 1 2 3   diadochokinesis   0 1 2 3
   0 1 2 3   associated movements   0 1 2 3
   (diadochokinesis of   (diadochokinesis
   right hand)   of left hand)

Finger-nose Test

Eyes open

   0 1 2   tremor   0 1 2
   0 1 2   touching nose correctly   0 1 2
   yes   no   consistent deviation to left   yes   no
   yes   no   consistent deviation to right   yes   no

Eyes Closed

   0 1 2   tremor   0 1 2
   0 1 2   touching nose correctly   0 1 2
   yes   no   consistent deviation to left   yes   no
   yes   no   consistent deviation to right   yes   no

Fingertip-touching Test

Eyes open

   0 1 2   tremor during movement   0 1 2
   0 1 2   tremor in placed finger   0 1 2
   0 1 2   placing finger correctly   0 1 2
   yes   no   consistent deviation to left   yes   no
   yes   no   consistent deviation to right   yes   no

Eyes closed

   0 1 2   tremor during movement   0 1 2
   0 1 2   tremor in placed finger   0 1 2
   0 1 2   placing finger correctly   0 1 2
   yes   no   consistent deviation to left   yes   no
   yes   no   consistent deviation to right   yes   no

Finger Opposition Test

   0 1 2   smoothness   0 1 2
   0 1 2   finger-to-finger transition   0 1 2
   0 1 2   mirror movements   0 1 2

Standing with Eyes Closed

   balance   0 1 2 3
   tendency to fall consistently to the left, right side.

							State	Soc. Resp.

Posture

Head

	0	1	2	rotated	0	1	2	
	0	1	2	bent laterally	0	1	2	
(ante)	0	1	2	flexed	0	1	2	(retro)

Trunk

0	1	2	rotated	0	1	2
0	1	2	bent laterally	0	1	2
0	1	2	kyphosis	0	1	2
0	1	2	lordosis	0	1	2
		symmetrically collapsed	0	1	2

Arms

0	1	2	endorotation	0	1	2
0	1	2	exorotation	0	1	2
0	1	2	flexion	0	1	2
0	1	2	extension	0	1	2
0	1	2	adduction	0	1	2
0	1	2	abduction	0	1	2

Gait

				width (constancy)	0	1		
				(measurement)	0	1	2	3
0	1	2		circumduction	0	1	2	
0	1	2		movements of pelvis	0	1	2	
0	1	2		movements of knees	0	1	2	
0	1	2		heel-toe gait	0	1	2	
0	1	2	3	arm movements	0	1	2	3

Placing of Feet

0	1	2	abduction	0	1	2
0	1	2	adduction	0	1	2
0	1	2	dorsiflexion	0	1	2
0	1	2	plantar flexion	0	1	2
0	1	2	on medial side	0	1	2
0	1	2	on lateral side	0	1	2

Walking along a Straight Line

		0	1	2	3	4	deviations	0	1	2	3	4
		0	1	2	3	4	other gross motor deviations	0	1	2	3	4
			0	1	2	3	walking on tiptoe	0	1	2	3	
			0	1	2	3	associated movements	0	1	2	3	
			0	1	2	3	walking on heels	0	1	2	3	
			0	1	2	3	associated movements	0	1	2	3	
0	1	2	3	4	5	6	standing on one leg	0	1	2	3	4	5	6
0	1	2	3	4	5	6	hopping	0	1	2	3	4	5	6

ASSESSMENT OF THE TRUNK

	State	Soc. Resp.

Inspection of the Back and Spine

0 = normal   5 = operation scars
1 = slight hairiness 6 = lipomas
2 = tufts of hair   7 = café-au-lait spots
3 = cutaneous dimples 8 = other: describe
4 = sinus opening

scoliosis to left   0   1   2
scoliosis to right   0   1   2
kyphosis   0   1   2
lordosis   0   1   2
limitation of movements: no
                                     yes (describe)

Skin Reflexes   abdominal skin reflex
0   1   2   supra-umbilical   0   1   2
0   1   2   umbilical   0   1   2
0   1   2   infra-umbilical   0   1   2

0   1   2   cremasteric reflex   0   1   2
0   1   2   Galant response   0   1   2

ASSESSMENT OF LYING

	State	Soc. Resp.

Prone

Spine   0   1   2   scoliosis   0   1   2
                        processi spinosi present
                                          absent (describe)
            limitation of movement no
                                    yes (describe)

For examination of hip joints, see page 94 of Proforma.

Posture of Legs and Feet in Prone Position
0   1   2   exorotation   0   1   2
0   1   2   abduction   0   1   2
0   1   2   adduction   0   1   2
0   1   2   flexion   0   1   2
0   1   2   extension   0   1   2
0   1   2   endorotation   0   1   2

Posture of Legs and Feet in Supine Position
0   1   2   abduction   0   1   2
0   1   2   adduction   0   1   2
0   1   2   flexion   0   1   2
0   1   2   extension   0   1   2
0   1   2   exorotation   0   1   2
0   1   2   endorotation   0   1   2

Knee-heel Test
0   1   2   accurate placing   0   1   2
0   1   2   sliding heel   0   1   2

Sitting up Without Help of Hands   0   1   2

99

ASSESSMENT OF THE HEAD

	State	Soc. Resp.

Facial Musculature

0	1	2	at rest	0	1	2
0	1	2	voluntary movements	0	1	2
0	1	2	emotional movements	0	1	2

Position of Eyes

no strabismus and no heterophoria
no strabismus, heterophoria
　　　　　exophoria　　left
　　　　　exophoria　　right
　　　　　hyperphoria　both
　　　　　hypophoria
concomitant strabismus
　　　　　convergent　left
　　　　　divergent　　right
　　　　　other　　　　both
non-concomitant strabismus (describe)

Fixation

deviation:　　　　　　　　　no
　　　　　　　　　　　　　　left, type:
　　　　　　　　　　　　　　right, type:
　　　　　　　　　　　　　　both, type:
choreiform movements:　　　absent
　　　　　　　　　　　　　　present
manifest strabismus:　　　　absent
　　　　　　　　　　　　　　present, type:

Pursuit Movements

range of movements　　　　intact
　　　　　　　　　　　　　　deviant (describe)
choreiform movements:　　　absent
　　　　　　　　　　　　　　present
ataxic eye movements:　　　absent
　　　　　　　　　　　　　　present
manifest strabismus:　　　　absent
　　　　　　　　　　　　　　present, type:

Convergence

left eye:	0	1	2
right eye:	0	1	2

pupillary reaction:　　　　absent
　　　　　　　　　　　　　present

Nystagmus

spontaneous nystagmus:　　absent
　　　　　　　　　　　　　present
direction:
intensity:
directional nystagmus:　　absent
　　　　　　　　　　　　　present
direction:
intensity:

	State	Soc. Resp.

Optokinetic Nystagmus
symmetrical
asymmetrical
vertical
horizontal

Pupillary Reactions
    direct: 0 1 2
    indirect: 0 1 2

Visual Acuity
    normal
    abnormal (specify)

Visual Field
    normal
    abnormal (specify)

Choreiform Movements of the Face
absent
present

Ears
    0 1 2   low voice   0 1 2
    0 1 2   localisation of sound 0 1 2

Tongue
    motility: smooth
                              awkward
    choreiform movements: absent
                              present
    fasciculations: absent
                              present

Pharyngeal Arches
symmetrical
asymmetrical
(describe)

Spontaneous Motility
decreased
the same
increased

Funduscopy
normal
abnormal (specify)

General Data

height:

weight:

circumference of skull:

abnormalities of skull:

general paediatric data:

preference of hands: right, left, both

preference of feet: right, left, both

preference of eyes: right, left, both

fine motor coordination in manipulation:

tactile sensation:

pain:

temperature:

kinesthesia:

sense of position:

dermographia:

speech:

REFERENCES

Abercrombie, M. L. J. (1968) 'Some notes on spatial disability: movement, intelligence quotient and attentiveness.' *Develop. Med. Child Neurol.*, **10**, 206.
—— Lindon, R. L., Tyson, M. C. (1964) 'Associated movements in normal and physically handicapped children.' *Develop. Med. Child Neurol.*, **6**, 573.
Abrams, A. L. (1968) 'Delayed irregular maturation versus minimal brain injury. Recommendations for a change in current nomenclature.' *Clin. Pediat.*, **7**, 344.
Aigner, B. R., Siekert, R. G. (1959) 'Differential diagnosis of acute ataxia in children.' *Proc. Mayo Clin.*, **34**, 573.
Anderson, W. W. (1963) 'The hyperkinetic child; a neurological appraisal.' *Neurology (Minneap.)*, **13**, 968.
André-Thomas, S., Chesni, Y., Saint-Anne Dargassies, S. (1960) The Neurological Examination of the Infant. Little Club Clinics in Developmental Medicine No. 1. London: SIMP/Heinemann Medical.
Bakwin, H. (1967) 'Developmental hyperactivity.' *Acta paediat. scand.*, Suppl. 172, 25.
Bax, M., Mac Keith, R. (1963) Minimal Cerebral Dysfunction. Clinics in Developmental Medicine, No. 10. London: Spastics Society with Heinemann.
Bell, R. Q. (1969) 'Stimulus control of parent or caretaker behavior by offspring.' Paper read at the 76th Annual Convention of the American Psychological Association, Division of Developmental Psychology.
Belmont, I., Birch, H. G., Karp, E. (1966) 'The disordering of intersensory and intrasensory integration by brain damage.' *J. nerv. ment. Dis.*, **141**, 410.
Benjamin, R. M., Thompson, R. F. (1959) 'Differential effects of cortical lesions in infant and adult cats on roughness discrimination.' *Exp. Neurol.*, **1**, 305.
Bergès, J., Lézine, I. (1965) The Imitation of Gestures. Clinics in Developmental Medicine, No. 18. London: Spastics Society with Heinemann.
Birch, H. G., Belmont, I. (1965) 'Auditory-visual integration in brain-damaged and normal children.' *Develop. Med. Child Neurol.*, **7**, 135.
—— —— (1966) 'Development and disturbance in auditory visual integration.' *E.E.N.T. Dig.*, **28**, 47.
—— Bortner, M. (1967) 'Stimulus competition and concept utilization in brain damaged children.' *Develop. Med. Child Neurol.*, **9**, 402.
—— Thomas, A., Chess, S. (1964) 'Behavioral development in brain damaged children.' *Arch. gen. Psychiat.*, **11**, 596.
Brenner, M. W., Gillman, S., Zangwill, O. L., Farrell, M. (1967) 'Visuo-motor disability in schoolchildren.' *Brit. med. J.*, **4**, 259.
Clements, S. D. (1962) 'Minimal brain dysfunction in the school-age child.' *Arch. gen. Psychiat.*, **6**, 185.
—— (1966) 'The child with minimal brain dysfunction.' *J. Lancet*, **86**, 121.
Cohen, H. J., Taft, L. T., Mahadeviah, M. S., Birch, H. G. (1967) 'Developmental changes in overflow in normal and aberrantly functioning children.' *J. Pediat.*, **71**, 39.
Conners, C. K. (1967) 'The syndrome of minimal brain dysfunction: psychological aspects.' *Pediat. Clin. N. Amer.*, **14**, 749.
Connolly, K., Stratton, P. (1968) 'Developmental changes in associated movements.' *Develop. Med. Child Neurol.*, **10**, 49.
Dobbing, J. (1968) 'Vulnerable periods in developing brain.' *in* Davison, A. N., Dobbing, J. (Eds.) Applied Neurochemistry. Oxford: Blackwell. p. 287.
Eisenberg, L. (1966) 'The management of the hyperkinetic child.' *Develop. Med. Child Neurol.*, **8**, 593.
Fog, E., Fog, M. (1963) 'Cerebral inhibition examined by associated movements.' *in* Bax, M., Mac Keith, R. *Loc. cit.*, p. 52.
Francis-Williams, J. (1963) 'Problems of development in children with 'minimal brain damage'.' *in* Bax, M., Mac Keith, R. *Loc. cit.*, p. 39.
Goldstein, K. (1936) 'Modifications of behavior consequent to cerebral lesions.' *Psychiat. Quart.*, **10**, 586.
Gomez, B. M. R. (1967) 'Minimal cerebral dysfunction (maximal neurologic confusion).' *Clin. Pediat.*, **6**, 589.
Graham, P., Rutter, M. (1968) 'Organic brain dysfunction and child psychiatric disorder.' *Brit. med. J.*, **3**, 695.
Gubbay, S. S., Ellis, E., Walton, J. N., Court, S. D. M. (1965) 'Clumsy children, a study of apraxic and agnosic defects in 21 children.' *Brain*, **88**, 295.
Hart de Ruyter, T. (1961) 'De psychische ontwikkeling van kinderen met lichte hersenbeschadigingen.' *Ned. Tijdschr. Geneesk.*, **105**, 745.
Holt, K. S. (1965) Assessment of Cerebral Palsy. London: Lloyd-Luke.

103

Illingworth, R. S. (1963) 'The clumsy child.' *in* Bax, M., Mac Keith, R. *Loc. cit.*, p. 26.
—— (1968) 'Delayed motor development.' *Pediat. Clin. N. Amer.*, **15**, 569.
Ingram, T. T. S. (1956) 'A characteristic form of overactive behaviour in brain damaged children.' *J. ment. Sci.*, **102**, 550.
—— (1963) 'Chronic brain syndromes in childhood other than cerebral palsy, epilepsy and mental defect.' *in* Bax, M., Mac Keith, R. *Loc. cit.*, p. 10.
—— (1966) 'The neurology of cerebral palsy.' *Arch. Dis. Childh.*, **41**, 337.
—— Stark, G. D., Blackburn, I. (1967) 'Ataxia and other neurological disorders as sequels of severe hypoglycaemia in childhood.' *Brain*, **90**, 851.
Kling, A. (1965) 'Behavioral and somatic development following lesions of the amygdala in the cat.' *J. psychiat. Res.*, **3**, 363.
—— (1966) 'Ontogenetic and phylogenetic studies on the amygdaloid nuclei.' *Psychosomat. Med.*, **28**, 155.
—— Tucker, T. J. (1968) 'Sparing of function following localized brain lesions in neonatal monkeys.' *in* Isaacson, R. L. (Ed.) The Neuropsychology of Development. New York: John Wiley. p. 121.
Knobloch, H., Pasamanick, B. (1959) 'The syndrome of minimal cerebral damage in infancy.' *J. Amer. med. Ass.*, **170**, 1384.
Köng, E. (1963) 'Minimal cerebral palsy: the importance of its recognition.' *in* Bax, M., Mac Keith R. *Loc. cit.*, p. 29.
Mac Keith, R. (1963) 'Defining the concept of "minimal brain damage".' *in* Bax, M., Mac Keith, R. *Loc. cit.*, p. 1.
McFie, J. (1963) 'An introduction to the problem of "minimal brain damage".' *in* Bax, M., Mac Keith, R. *Loc. cit.*, p. 18
Millichap, J. G. (1968) 'Drugs in management of hyperkinetic and perceptually handicapped children.' *J. Amer. med. Ass.*, **206**, 1527.
Minde, K., Webb, G., Sykes, D. (1968) 'Studies on the hyperactive child. VI. Prenatal and paranatal factors associated with hyperactivity.' *Develop. Med. Child Neurol.*, **10**, 355.
Müller, D. (1968) Neurologische Untersuchung und Diagnostik im Kindesalter. Wien: Springer.
Munsat, T. L., Pearson, C. M. (1967) 'The differential diagnosis of neuromuscular weakness in infancy and childhood. I. Non-dystrophic disorders.' *Develop. Med. Child Neurol.*, **9**, 220.
Osofsky, H. J. (1969) 'Antenatal malnutrition: its relationship to subsequent infant and child development.' *Amer. J. Obstet. Gynec.*, **105**, 1150.
Paine, R. S. (1966) 'Neurological grand rounds: minimal chronic brain syndromes.' *Clin. Proc. Child Hosp. D.C.*, **22**, 21.
—— Oppé, T. E. (1966) Neurological Examination of Children. Clinics in Developmental Medicine, Nos. 21/22. London: Spastics Society with Heinemann.
—— Werry, J. S., Quay, H. C. (1968) 'A study "minimal cerebral dysfunction".' *Develop. Med. Child Neurol.*, **10**, 505.
Pincus, J. H., Glaser, G. H. (1966) 'The syndrome of "minimal brain damage" in childhood.' *New Engl. J. Med.*, **275**, 27.
Pond, D. (1960) 'Is there a syndrome of "brain damage" in children?'. *Cerebr. Palsy Bull.*, **2**, 296.
Prechtl, H. F. R. (1963) 'The mother-child interaction in babies with minimal brain damage.' *in* Foss, B. M. (Ed.) Determinants of Infant Behaviour. Vol. II. London: Methuen. p. 53.
—— (1965) 'Prognostic value of neurological signs in the newborn infant.' *Proc. roy. Soc. Med.*, **58**, 3.
—— Beintema, D. J. (1964) The Neurological Examination of the Full-Term Newborn Infant. Clinics in Developmental Medicine, No. 12. London: Spastics Society with Heinemann.
—— Lenard, H. G. (1968) 'Verhaltensphysiologie des Neugeborenen.' *in* Linneweh, F. (Ed.) Forstschritte Pädologie. Berlin: Springer.
—— Stemmer, C. (1962) 'The choreiform syndrome in children.' *Develop. Med. Child Neurol.*, **4**, 119.
Reuben, R. N., Bakwin, H. (1968) 'Developmental clumsiness.' *Pediat. Clin. N. Amer.*, **15**, 601.
Robson, P. (1968) 'Persisting head turning in the early months: some effects in the early years.' *Develop. Med. Child Neurol.*, **10**, 82.
Rutter, M., Graham, P., Birch, H. G. (1966) 'Interrelations between the choreiform syndrome, reading disability and psychiatric disorder in children of 8-11 years.' *Develop. Med. Child Neurol.*, **8**, 149.
—— Graham, P., Yule, W. (1970) A Neuropsychiatric Study in Childhood. Clinics in Developmental Medicine No. 35/36. London: Spastics Society with Heinemann Medical; Philadelphia: J. B. Lippincott.
Sainz, A. (1966) 'Hyperkinetic disease of children: diagnosis and therapy.' *Dis. nerv. Syst.*, **27**, 48.
Schain, R. J. (1970) 'Neurological evaluation of children with learning disorders.' *Neuropädiatrie*, **1**, 307.
Scharlock, D. P., Tucker, T. J., Strominger, N. L. (1963) 'Auditory discrimination by the cat after neonatal ablation of temporal cortex.' *Science*, **141**, 1197.
Schwartz, N. B., Kling, A. (1964) 'The effect of amygdaloid lesions on feeding, grooming and reproduction in rats.' *Acta neuroveg.*, **26**, 12.

Sheridan, M. D. (1969) 'The development of vision, hearing and communication in babies and young children.' *Proc. roy. Soc. Med.*, **62**, 999.

Skatveldt, M. (1963) 'Minimal brain damage.' *in* Bax, M., Mac Keith, R. *Loc. cit.*, p. 32.

Stemmer, C. (1964) Choreiforme bewegingsonrust (een oriënterend onderzoek). Thesis: Groningen.

Stevens, D. A., Boydstun, J. A., Dijkman, R. A., Peters, J. E., Sinton, D. W. (1967) 'Presumed minimal brain dysfunction in children.' *Arch. gen. Psychiat.*, **16**, 281.

Stewart, M. A., Pitts, F. W., Craig, A. G., Dieruf, W. (1966) 'The hyperactive child syndrome.' *Amer. J. Orthopsychiat.*, **34**, 861.

Strauss, A. A., Werner, H. (1943) 'Comparative psychopathology of brain-injured child and traumatic brain-injured adult.' *Amer. J. Psychiat.*, **99**, 835.

Stutte, H. (1966) 'Das zerebral geschädigte Kind.' *Therapiewoche*, **16**, 1499.

Tardieu, G. (1968) Infirmités Motrices Cérébrales. *Rev. Neuropsychiat. infant.*, **16**, No. 1-2.

Thompson, C. I., Schwartzbaum, J. S., Harlow, H. F. (1969) 'Development of social fear after amygalectomy in infant rhesus monkeys.' *Physiol. Behav.*, **4**, 249.

Tucker, T. J., Kling, A. (1969) 'Preservation of delayed response following combined lesions of prefrontal and posterior association cortex in infant monkeys.' *Exp. Neurol.*, **23**, 491.

Walker, M. (1965) 'Perceptual, coding, visuo-motor and spatial difficulties and their neurological correlates.' *Develop. Med. Child Neurol.*, **7**, 543.

Walton, J. N. (1963) 'Clumsy children.' *in* Bax, M., Mac Keith, R. *Loc. cit.*, p. 24.

—— Ellis, E., Court, S. D. M. (1962) 'Clumsy children: developmental apraxia and agnosia.' *Brain*, **85**, 603.

Werry, J. S. (1968) 'Studies on the hyperactive child. IV. An empirical analysis of the minimal brain dysfunction syndrome.' *Arch. gen. Psychiat.*, **19**, 9.

—— Weiss, G., Douglas, V. (1964) 'Studies on the hyperactive child. I. Some preliminary findings.' *Canad. Psychiat. Ass. J.*, **9**, 120.

Wetzel, A. B., Thompson, V. E., Horel, J. A., Meyer, P. M. (1965) 'Some consequences of perinatal lesions of the visual cortex in the cat.' *Psychon. Sci.*, **3**, 381.

Wigglesworth, R. (1961) 'Minimal cerebral palsy.' *Cerebr. Palsy Bull.*, **3**, 293.

—— (1963) 'The importance of recognising minimal cerebral dysfunction in paediatric practice.' *in* Bax, M., Mac Keith, R. *Loc. cit.*, p. 34.

Winick, M. (1969) 'Malnutrition and brain development.' *J. Pediat.*, **74**, 667.

Wolff, P. H., Hurwitz, I. (1966) 'The choreiform syndrome.' *Develop. Med. Child Neurol.*, **8**, 160.

Work, H. H., Haldane, J. E. (1966) 'Cerebral dysfunction in children.' *Amer. J. Dis. Child.*, **111**, 573.

Zazzo, R., (Ed.) (1960) Manuel pour l'Examination Psychologique de l'Enfant. Neuchâtel: De la Chaux & Niestlé.